THE ESSENTIAL GUIDE TO DENTAL IMPLANTS

BY DR ANDREA UBHI

BCHD

WITH DR ADAM GLASSFORD

BCHD DIP CON SED(NCLE) DIP IMP DENT
(RCS)(ENG.)(ADV CERT)

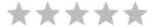

"In this guide, Andrea brings practical and insightful advice, and simplifies a seemingly complex subject."

Elle Jasleen

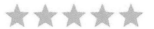

"Want to know about implants? Then start with this book. It is a road map, navigating this advanced world of modern dentistry."

Matthew Daljit

"I loved reading a no-nonsense surgeon's perspective. Made perfect sense to me."

Paul Dixon

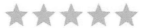

"A fantastic read and a great insight into the world of implants!"

Zoe Gilroy

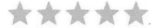

"This book has totally changed my thinking. I thought it wasn't relevant to me. It is relevant to everyone. This book holds an energy and passion."

Paul Thorpe

"The book is amazing!! It covers everything you need to know about treatment. Everyone should read this."

Ric Fisher

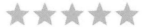

"This message matters deeply and is relevant for every person in the world. I'm shocked by some of the facts I never knew. Now I do and it will change my future."

Nicholas Jagar

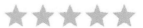

"This book is smart and honest. No holds barred."

Rosemary Taylor

The information contained in this book is for general educational purposes only. It is not intended and should not be relied on as dental advice. The authors are not responsible for any specific dental health need that requires dental supervision. You should contact a qualified dental professional for appropriate personal advice.

ISBN 978-1-9162400-0-1

TO OUR PATIENTS

For sharing your journey with us. Thank
you for inspiring us to write this book to
share the great secret.

TO OUR TEAM

For your support and honesty. Thank you
for encouraging us to strive for excellence
every single day.

TO OUR REFERRING DENTISTS

For your trust in us.

CONTENTS

INTRODUCTION

"A smile makes the world a beautiful place. When you lose your smile, you lose your way in the chaos of life."

ROY T. BENNETT

INTRODUCTION

Imagine smiling the most beautiful and confident smile. Picture biting into crisp apples. Imagine laughing uncontrollably, showing off dazzling, secure teeth. Imagine no more dentures.

As you read this book, you will become equipped with the knowledge to make lifechanging decisions about failing or missing teeth, or about loose dentures.

You will feel hope.

First, let me tell you a story.

A few years ago, a concerned daughter asked if I would look at her ageing mother and see if there was anything I could do with her mother's loose dentures.

Her mother wasn't eating and her daughter was worried. Her mother had lost her teeth one by one over the years. After each tooth had been lost, a new partial denture had been made. Finally, all her teeth had been lost, and she was given full dentures. That was over 20 years ago.

Every new set of dentures felt looser and more uncomfortable than the previous set.

The bone had shrunk dramatically after the teeth had been lost. Her dentures were simply balancing on her jaws, pressing directly onto the nerves that lie just under the gums. She had to bite very gently or she experienced pain.

As this lady tried to talk to me at the consultation, she struggled so much to control her loose dentures. She told me that she could not bite or chew. She was only able to drink blended foods, which she hated, and she was taking multiple medications for indigestion. She was struggling to maintain a well-balanced diet and the nutrition she needed. Month by month, year by year, she had been weakening.

Imagine there is a breakthrough treatment that could replace missing and failing teeth with something so similar to your natural teeth that you could bite and chew anything you want to. Imagine being able to live and laugh freely without worry? Would you be interested?

Well this lady certainly was.

It is time for a second chance at having healthy teeth.

Imagine the possibilities.

SECTION 1

THE REALITY OF MISSING TEETH

"Do you know what is the real price of having missing teeth? Few people do."

THE OVERWHELMING EPIDEMIC

THE PSYCHOLOGICAL PRICE OF TOOTH LOSS

To me, having teeth extracted just seems barbaric in this modern world of fast-paced science, and I guess you feel the same.

I remember the first tooth I saw being taken out when I was training at dental school. Quite honestly, I was shocked. I didn't realise that kind of thing really happened.

I was astonished at the numbers of teeth being taken out. Thousands. Hundreds of thousands.

We are still a really long way away from a world of perfect teeth for life.

I've been looking at statistics about tooth loss. In the UK, each adult on average has lost 6 teeth each.

Unbelievable.

Listen to this, an enormous 6% of the population in England, Wales and Northern Ireland have no teeth whatsoever! This means that 2.7 million of all these adults are struggling with no teeth at all (*The 2009 Adult Dental Health Survey*).

This is an epidemic.

Let's take a big step back.

If you have a problem with a tooth, then there are two different solutions – if possible, get it fixed, or have the tooth taken out.

One of the first questions we get asked as dentists at this decisive moment is, "How much is it to fix the tooth or how much to take it out?"

However, there isn't a simple price comparison. There are much more important issues at stake.

Life will NOT be simpler or cheaper after an extraction.

Trust me.

As you read on, you will be amazed at the significant evidence we will present you with.

Do you know what is the real price of having missing teeth?

Think about it.

Probably not. Few people do.

Well, we are going to tell you.

A friend of ours, Rob Keating, tells this story.

> "When I was 23, I broke one of my back teeth on a hard sweet when I was in Australia. I was there for a year and didn't have dental health insurance, so I didn't go to the dentist. I just lived with a broken tooth for that year.
>
> When I got back to the UK, I went straight to my dentist. I needed root treatment and he gave me a crown. It lasted 15 years.
>
> Then all of a sudden, I got an infection. My face was swollen and massive! It was an absolute nightmare. They tried to treat it with antibiotics, but it was so painful that I just had the tooth out.
>
> My wife said just leave the space, as no one could see it. I left it a while. But in a matter of weeks, I felt my other teeth shifting. Literally in a matter of weeks! Where my other teeth had been so tight together and I could barely get the floss down, all of a sudden there were big gaps and I had to use big brushes between my teeth instead of floss. And where the tooth had been taken out, the bone recession was enormous!
>
> It was the first tooth that I had lost. All of a sudden, I felt like I'm getting old. I'm almost 40. I have this thing that has been taken away from me that will never grow back. Nothing like this has ever happened to me before in my life."

We are going to hear the rest of Rob's story later, but first let's look at some statistics.

According to a study by the American Association of Cosmetic Dentistry (2004)

"99.7% of people believe that a smile is an important social asset"

If we have missing teeth, like it or not, we are judged.

SOCIAL STIGMA

One man came to us for help. He told us that he was getting depressed.

A few years ago, he had had a significant accident and sadly, he had lost one of his front teeth. He'd tried a denture to fill the gap, but just couldn't get used to it as it made him feel sick. So, he just lived with the gap in his smile.

However, not long after the accident, he went to a pub with his friends and the doorman refused him entry, as he considered this lovely man to look too rough for the establishment!

This engaging man stopped going out.

Having missing teeth affects how we are perceived socially. And this affects our confidence.

BEREAVEMENT

A desperate lady wrote an email to our team just a few weeks ago. She simply said, "Please help. I've just had my front tooth out. I'm devastated. I won't leave the house. I feel mortified. Please can you help me?"

If you have had experience of tooth loss, then you probably know this. When we lose a tooth, particularly a front tooth, there can be a feeling of emotional loss that is similar to losing something or someone precious in our lives forever. Losing a tooth is irreversible. Not only can there be acute embarrassment that brings with it a deep lack of confidence, also there can be a long period of mourning.

We all know that confidence is a fragile thing. Some of the most beautiful moments in life are when we openly smile, laugh and talk.

When we smile, people reciprocate and smile back at us.

Imagine this. If we are embarrassed of our smiles, ashamed of missing teeth or terrified that our dentures might fall out, then we close our lips, we cover our mouths, we hide our faces with our hands and we shut down. We stop laughing. We pull back socially. We become introverted or appear so.

Those around us may take this social 'pulling back' as a signal that we don't want to communicate, or at worst, that we dislike them and are being hostile.

Let's be honest with ourselves here, it is our missing teeth and loose dentures that are holding us back and putting us into social isolation.

LACK OF CONFIDENCE
A few years ago, I was delighted to be invited to the wedding of my friends. The couple were radiant and looked beautiful.

I stood behind the official photographer as he was taking an enormous bridal party photo. As he went to capture the photo, he shouted, "Say cheese!" As I watched, imagine my surprise when I saw almost 50% of this big group clamping their lips tightly shut for the camera, whereas the other 50% dazzled their teeth for the photo. Now, as a dentist, I was intrigued. So, I spent the rest of the day chatting to as many people as I possibly could and analysing the different smiles of both groups.

What I found was really interesting. The ones who closed their lips together for the photograph, all had aesthetic issues with their smiles. I could see dentures, missing teeth, discoloured fillings, ugly crowns or crooked teeth. Interestingly, even during simple conversation, many of this group put their hand over their mouths when chatting and smiling.

They were demonstrating what we call a low level of 'Smiling Confidence.'

However, the ones from the other group, the ones who smiled broadly and confidently for the photo, typically had great teeth and showed a very high level of 'Smiling Confidence.'

Next time you are at a wedding and there is a group photo, stand behind the photographer and see for yourself.

Try this easy questionnaire to assess your own level of 'Smiling Confidence.'

THE SMILING CONFIDENCE TEST

1. When smiling, do you

    a. normally show off your teeth?

    b. close your mouth?

2. After a meal

    a. are you normally confident your teeth will be clean?

    b. are you worried that you will have food stuck between your teeth?

3. Look at several photographs of yourself, do you

    a. normally show your teeth when smiling?

    b. do you rarely show your teeth?

4. When laughing, do you

    a. normally laugh freely?

    b. usually put your hand over your mouth?

5. When talking with people close up, do you normally

    a. feel proud and confident of your smile?

    b. normally feel self-conscious?

Count up the number of questions that you answered as an (a):

> 0 = No Smiling Confidence at all
>
> 1 = Very low Smiling Confidence
>
> 2 = Low Smiling Confidence
>
> 3 = Mediocre Smiling Confidence
>
> 4 = Reasonably high Smiling Confidence.
>
> 5 =Total Smiling Confidence. Dazzle the world with your smile!

If we go through life pulling back from social interactions and reducing our smiling, then people may misinterpret this. They may think that we do not like them or that we have something to hide, and pull back from us. This is a Catch 22 situation.

Consider this.

Having beautiful teeth may not actually make you happier in itself, however having beautiful teeth increases our 'Smiling Confidence.' And as we smile more openly and freely, then due to social reciprocation, people smile back at us. So, we smile more at them and they smile more at us.

You understand the point.

We have listened to hundreds and hundreds of patients' before and after stories of their Smile Transformation journeys. I am a cosmetic dentistry patient, myself, I have to say, yes, having a beautiful smile does make us happier and makes those around us happier too.

Do you want a more beautiful, confident smile? Then keep reading. I think you will be interested, but first let's look at this question. Can missing teeth hinder our careers?

Imagine that you are an employer and that you are interviewing these two applicants in the following photos.

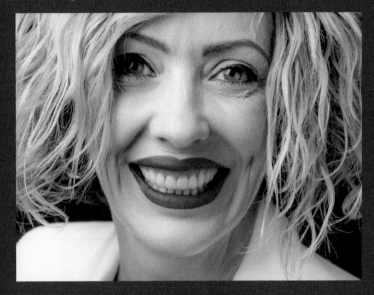

Applicant 1

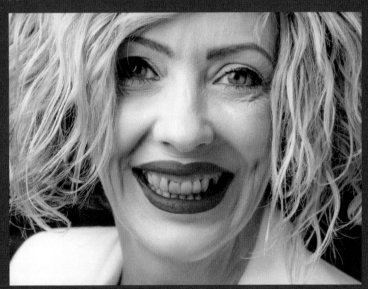

Applicant 2

Which version of me would you choose to employ?

Imagine at the interview, would you assess these two people the same? Would you equally want either candidate representing your company?

Remember, they are groomed the same, they have the same education and experience and it is the same person underneath the smile, with the same intelligence.

They have the same personality – or would they? Would both versions of me have the same confidence? I doubt it.

"74% of adults believe that an unattractive smile can hinder career success"

The American Academy of Cosmetic Dentistry 2004 Study.

A smile has power.

If you have missing teeth and want to be successful in your career, then you are going to be glued to the rest of this book.

Yes, losing teeth can affect your psychological well-being, your relationships and your career, however, can it affect us physically?

THE PHYSICAL PRICE OF TOOTH LOSS

Remember Rob's story? You may think like he initially did, that losing just one tooth isn't going to cause any problems.

However, if you have one tooth extracted, does that have an impact on the others around it?

Let's look at this revealing example. Imagine one of your molars is lost. Perhaps you're thinking that's no big deal, right?

Well, picture what can happen next.

DECAY AND GUM DISEASE

Over time, the teeth either side of the missing tooth can drift into the new space, just like Rob's did. The spaces opened up really quickly over the following few days after his tooth was removed.

This immediately causes food to become trapped between the teeth when eating and can be uncomfortable. Bigger spaces between your teeth are more difficult to clean.

What do you think happens then?

There is an increased risk of decay and gum disease.

Now keep reading, as there is more.

When a tooth has been removed, the bone shrinks back *quickly and irreversibly*. In the first 6 months after tooth extraction, most bone loss occurs and then *continues indefinitely*.

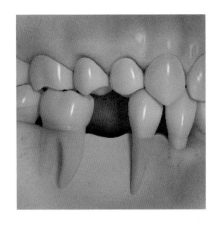

A tooth recently removed.

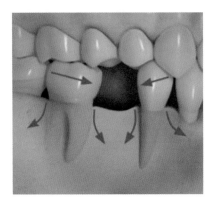

The adjacent teeth start drifting into the space and the bone starts shrinking back.

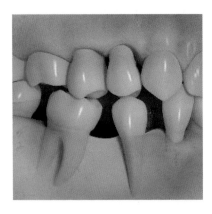

The teeth above the space may start drifting downwards into the new space.

The bone can also shrink from the sides of the remaining teeth that are adjacent to the space too. This causes accelerated gum recession and the root surface is exposed. This soft and extremely vulnerable root surface is called *cementum*.

Cementum is much, much softer than enamel and highly prone to decay, causing *root cavities*. The distance from the cementum surface to the nerve inside the tooth is just a few millimetres, so decay can reach the nerve of the tooth super-quick, way quicker than decay passing through enamel. If decay reaches the nerve, then infection can occur, which may result in an abscess. At this stage, the tooth will need to be treated with a root canal or be extracted.

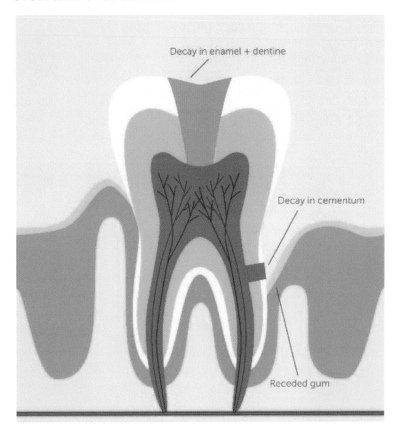

Decay in enamel + dentine

Decay in cementum

Receded gum

There is now an increased risk of losing a second tooth, then another and another.

OVER-ERUPTION

Now listen to this, where there is a missing *lower* tooth, then the teeth *above* the space often move downwards over time. And if there is a missing *upper* tooth, then the teeth below can move upwards into the space.

Why?

When there is no opposing force on a tooth, then the natural tendency is for the tooth to erupt further, becoming vertically out of line. Normally teeth bite together and exert opposing forces, keeping both upper and lower teeth in position.

Is this a problem?

INCREASED RISK OF TOOTH FRACTURE

Well yes, teeth that have 'over-erupted,' drifting into the space below or above, interfere with the way your jaw moves normally. As your jaw slides forwards, backwards and side to side, the 'over-erupted' teeth can get knocked in the powerful biting motion of the jaw. Over time, this can have an effect on the TMJ, the temporomandibular joint, causing significant pain. Also, the teeth that are getting knocked can loosen, become painful or suddenly fracture. These teeth are at much higher risk of tooth loss than before.

INCREASED WEAR

When you have all your natural teeth, the chewing forces are shared out relatively evenly over your lifetime. Normally, your teeth wear down at an even slow rate.

Now imagine that you have lost one tooth. That's one less tooth to share the load and forces of chewing. One missing tooth may not make a lot of difference, but over a lifetime, there will be a little more additional wear on the remaining teeth.

Now imagine that you have lost many teeth. Over a life-time, the increased forces on the remaining teeth can result in accelerated wear. Have a look at the photo below. This patient had lost many of the back teeth, so was using the front teeth to do most of the chewing. The front teeth became overloaded and the result was severe wear.

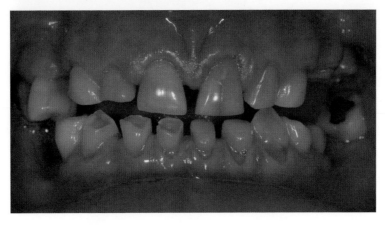

A patient with many missing back teeth and showing accelerated tooth wear on the remaining teeth.

Tooth wear is a common problem.

"77% of adults with teeth show some tooth wear in their front teeth"

Adult Dental Health Survey 2009

Losing teeth increases the wear on the remaining teeth.

More Chin, Less Height

'Face height' is the overall measurement of your face, and it is generally thought that when a face presents in equal thirds, then it is well-proportioned.

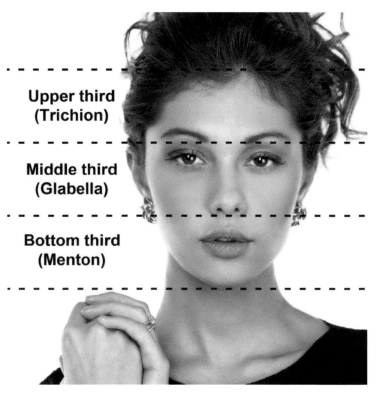

**Upper third
(Trichion)**

**Middle third
(Glabella)**

**Bottom third
(Menton)**

As a result of the tooth wear, there is a reduction of the face height one millimetre at a time. As you lose more teeth, then tooth wear is accelerated further. You can guess how this affects the appearance of the face overall.

Much more significantly, if you were to lose all your teeth, then the face height in the lower third of your face is reduced by up to 40mm. Measure that on your face. That is almost the whole height of your lower jaw!

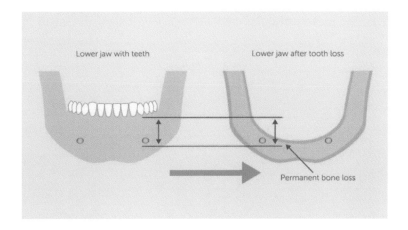

Lower jaw with teeth

Lower jaw after tooth loss

Permanent bone loss

Less Support Increases Wrinkles

As the jaw over-closes, it swings forwards, creating the 'Witch-Look.'

Not only does the vertical face height reduce, but also the width of the face reduces as there is reduced support from the teeth and bone, causing a hollowed appearance.

In a nutshell, this has a dramatic effect on your skin.

The skin is 'draped' over your bones and muscles.

Where there is reduced bone volume and less teeth to support the bone and skin, then the skin creases together in wide folds. Deep wrinkles develop from the nose to the corners of the mouth (*nasio-labial folds*) and from the corners of the mouth down to the jaw (*marionette lines*).

Imagine if you were unfortunate enough to have lost all your teeth in the upper or lower jaw or even both, then there is a significant reduction in both the face height and width.

Losing teeth can significantly increase wrinkles, as seen in these photos below.

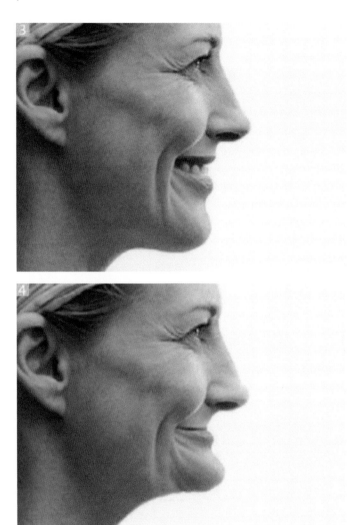

A LITTLE LESS POUT

The lips are supported by the teeth and underlying bone.

Take a look at the people around you. Look at people with naturally full, thick lips, and notice that their underlying teeth are prominent and full. This is particularly noticeable in people with protruding teeth. They often have gorgeous, full lips.

Now notice the people who have thin lips. Their teeth are set back and small.

Also notice those with asymmetry of the lips, and see how the teeth underlying are asymmetrical with some set out and some set back. This reflects how the lips are supported by the underlying structures.

Then see if you can spot some people with ultra-thin lips or even with no lips showing at all. You are probably looking at a person with no teeth at all and with significant bone shrinkage.

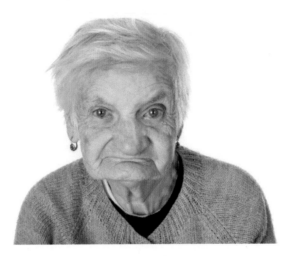

Note in the photo how this lady's lips are very thin, reflecting the lack of teeth in either one or both of the jaws. The jaws are 'over closing,' causing the lower jaw to swing forwards and be more prominent than the upper.

We have patients attending our clinic who ask for wrinkle-reduction procedures and lip fillers. However, often what these patients need foremost are reconstructive dental procedures to rebuild the face height and width of their jaws. The outcome of these treatments is far more effective than any facelift that I have ever seen.

It is amazing!

After the dental reconstruction, any remaining wrinkles or areas of low facial volume can then be treated with modern wrinkle procedures.

Losing teeth affects the way we look, but how does it affect our ability to bite and chew?

A Lot Less Bite

Have you ever noticed when you are out for dinner that you or others at the table are taking a long time looking over the menu, looking for foods that you *can eat, rather than ones that you want to eat*? People with missing teeth and dentures often need softer foods or foods cut into very small pieces so they are able to tackle them.

The difficulty of being able to bite and chew adequately is perhaps the most significant problem of losing teeth.

And there is research to prove this.

"Denture wearers have only about 20-25% of the total biting strength and chewing force of people with natural teeth [1]"

Full denture wearers need to chew their food approximately 7 times more than those with natural teeth.

Exhausting.

No wonder denture wearers choose softer foods that can be sucked rather than chewed.[2]

Losing teeth affects eating significantly. But does this have any impact on our overall health?

REDUCED NUTRITION

Research shows that tooth loss *does* have a negative impact on diet and the foods that we can choose.[3] [4]

Patients with all their teeth missing eat less fruits, vegetables and fibre. And they eat more cholesterol and saturated fats. This is an important development, as this increases the risk of obesity and can increase the risk of cardiovascular diseases and gut disorders.[5]

A great diet is made up of fresh fruits, vegetables, nuts, seeds and with loads of fibre. However, these foods are a challenge to bite and chew.

Research also showed that of older people who were missing all their teeth:

39% were prevented from eating foods they would like to eat.

29% reported a decline in their enjoyment of food.

14% avoided eating with others.[6]

Now we are coming to a really important part.

What you are going to learn next could seriously affect how long you live.

AN INCREASE IN DISEASES

Tooth loss can affect our general health in many different ways, let's look at the research.

When we have missing teeth, we may suffer from:

1. increased risk of gut diseases, including an increased rate of chronic inflammatory changes of the gastric mucosa, upper gastrointestinal and pancreatic cancer, and higher rates of peptic or duodenal ulcers.[7][8][9]
2. increased risk of Diabetes Type 2 [10][11]
3. increased risk of heart disease, hypertension, heart failure, ischaemic heart disease, stroke, and aortic valve sclerosis [12][13][14][15][16]
4. decreased daily function, physical activity, and the physical part of health-related quality of life [17][18]
5. increased risk of chronic kidney disease [19]
6. increased risk of sleep-disordered breathing, including obstructive sleep apnoea [20]
7. increased oral thrush and traumatic ulcers [21][22][23]

Having missing teeth is a serious and urgent health issue.

But first, let's go back to basics.

WHY DO WE LOSE TEETH?

I believe that the biggest cause of tooth loss is lack of knowledge. With knowledge right from the very beginning, we can learn how to keep our teeth for life.

Have you ever noticed that most dentists have great teeth for life? Interesting isn't it?

What do dentists know that the majority of the population doesn't?

Let's consider the four main causes of tooth loss to understand:

1. Decay
2. Fracture
3. Gum disease
4. Trauma

DECAY

First, what causes tooth decay?

Plaque is the white, sticky film that builds up on our teeth when we don't clean our teeth for several hours. Plaque contains bacteria. When these bacteria are fed with sugars and carbohydrates from our diets, they turn the plaque into acids. These acids cause decay (holes) in the teeth.

Eating and drinking too much acidic foods and drinks also causes decay and damage to our teeth too, even if we brush our teeth really well.

Decay normally needs treatment by your dentist. The decay is removed and the structure rebuilt with a dental filling material.

Decay is stopped in its tracks.

Now, as dentists, we love natural teeth. We will do everything that we possibly can to save teeth. Why?

Natural teeth are beautiful. They can feel temperature and give us more sensation when eating and drinking. When we bite, we can feel pressure through the nerves around the root, so we can feel how much force to use without damaging or breaking our teeth. Let's love our precious teeth and care for them carefully.

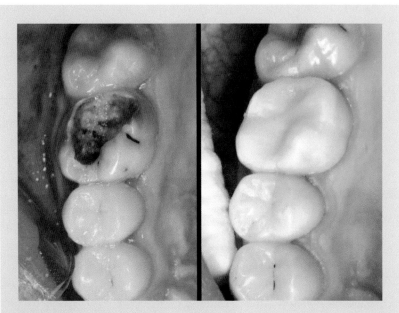

Before: decayed tooth.

After: decay removed and the hole repaired with a tooth coloured filling.

However, what happens if decay is left untreated?

Then there is a different ending to the story.

The decay becomes deeper and deeper, spreading to the very heart of the tooth where the nerve lies. This can result in severe pain, infection and an abscess. Untreated infected teeth can, on occasion, form an extra-oral sinus tract that can lead to permanent facial scarring.

If caught in time, then infected teeth can be treated with root canal treatment. Take a look at the diagram below. Under local anaesthetic, the infected nerve is removed, a filling is put into the centre of the tooth and then the tooth is rebuilt with a very large filling or crown.

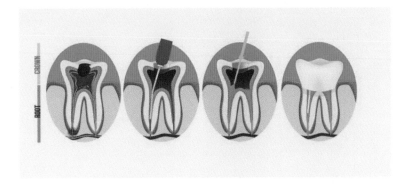

Diagram of the stages of root treatment: (1) infection of the root canal (2) cleaning the canal (3) filling the canal (4) restoring the molar tooth with a crown.

On the other hand, if too much enamel and dentine has been destroyed, then it may be too late for root treatment. The whole tooth needs to be extracted as soon as possible before infection spreads to your whole body and worst-case scenario, leads to life-threatening septicaemia.

REAL EXAMPLE

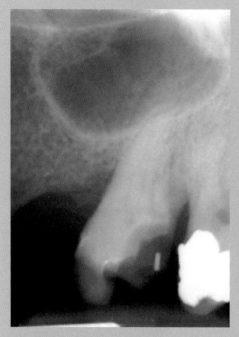

Before X-ray: a molar tooth which has decay to the nerve, causing symptoms including pain.

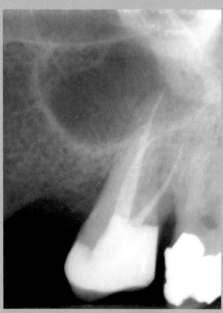

After X-ray: after root canal treatment and repair of the tooth crown.

Case by Dr Tim Steel, Andrea Ubhi Dentistry.

FRACTURE

Let's look at another reason that teeth are lost, and you may not have heard of this one.

If the front teeth wear down over time, as they commonly do, then increased forces are transferred to the back teeth as we bite and chew. These forces can be so high that they can overload the back teeth, sometimes causing whole tooth cusps to break off. However sometimes these high forces cause hairline fractures in the enamel that run vertically through the tooth.

> "We, as dentists, call this 'Cracked Tooth Syndrome.' This can be very difficult to diagnose. These hairline fractures can allow bacteria into the centre of the tooth, irritate the nerve, and may eventually lead to nerve death."
>
> Dr Tim Steel.

Treatment can involve root canal treatment, followed by a crown. Why have a crown? The crown splints the tooth walls together to prevent further fracturing.

However sometimes these teeth cannot be saved and need extracting.

If your front teeth are wearing down, then it may be time to discuss this with a dentist with a special interest in treating wear, to avoid bigger problems in the future.

Here is an example of a young woman with significant wear on her front teeth.

REAL EXAMPLE 1

SEVERE WEAR OF THE TIPS AND FRONT SURFACES OF THE
TEETH

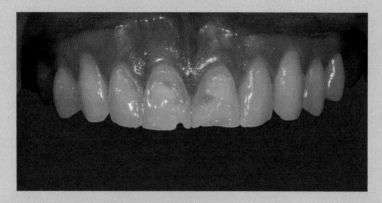

Before: Wear on the front teeth

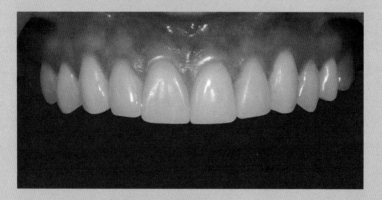

After: The wear has been treated with Composite Bonding.

Case by Dr Stephen Gibson, Andrea Ubhi Dentistry.

REAL EXAMPLE 2

SEVERE VERTICAL WEAR

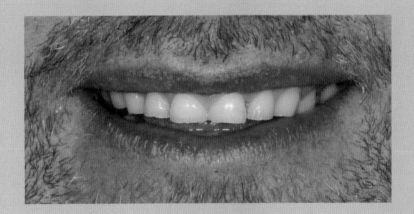

Before: Wear on the front teeth

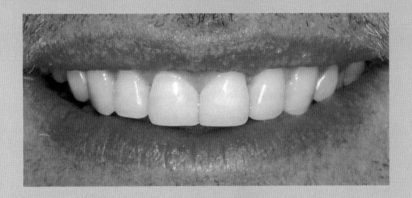

After: The wear has been treated with Composite Bonding.

Case by Dr Stephen Gibson, Andrea Ubhi Dentistry.

GUM DISEASE

Astonishingly, 83% of us who are adults have some gum disease, according to the 2009 Dental Health Survey.

And a massive 10-15% of the population will lose a significant number of teeth as a result of undiagnosed and untreated gum disease.

It is time to sit up and listen, so you can spot the signs of gum disease and get help and treatment you need!

In the diagram below, the gums and bone in the left side of the diagram are healthy, whereas the right side has gum disease. The diseased gums are swollen. The gums and bone are shrinking back. Eventually, there will be no support for the tooth, and the tooth will become loose and simply fall out.

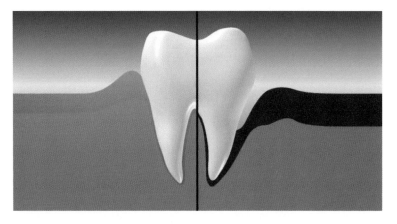

Have you ever heard stories of people taking out their own teeth? Well if you have no bone left around a tooth and it is hanging by a thread, then that's easy!

Remember, early diagnosis is so important. Early intervention simplifies treatment, improves prognosis and keeps your mouth fresh and healthy long term.

So, let's take a look at the signs.

THE EARLY WARNING SIGNS OF GUM DISEASE

The first sign is red and swollen gums which bleed after brushing or flossing. This is called *gingivitis*. This is a red alert warning.

Gingivitis is often the first stage of gum disease. Gingivitis is causes inflammation of the gums and is reversible.

Everyone gets bleeding gums, right? Everyone ignores it, don't they? Well since 83% of the population have gum disease, then there seems to be a lot of people doing just that.

Do not ignore bleeding gums!

Did you know that gingivitis is reversible?

Listen to what the hygienist at our practice, has to say.

"If you have bleeding gums this can be an indicator that you have the first stages of gum disease. This can be caused by not removing the soft plaque effectively from the teeth.
Plaque is made up from food debris and bacteria. Stain builds up from tea/coffee/smoking/red wine this increases the attraction of plaque to the tooth surface. You need to be brushing twice a day morning and night. However, a brush doesn't get in between your teeth very well. Interdental cleaning is really important to reach these difficult areas.

Ideally you should use a combination of both floss and interdental brushes.
If the soft plaque is not removed effectively within a period of 48 hours the soft plaque hardens into a deposit called calculus/tartar.
This needs to be removed by a hygienist, therapist or dentist.

If the calculus is left it can produce toxins and enzymes which destroy the supporting bone. There are lots of links between the effects of gum disease and other systemic conditions in the body including heart disease, diabetes, asthma.
Think about hygienist appointments as regular body maintenance appointments."

JENNIE SCOTT RDH

HYGIENIST AT ANDREA UBHI DENTISTRY

If you have bleeding gums, then this means that you are not cleaning your teeth absolutely perfectly. We have to clean our teeth 100% every day.

No exceptions.

So, brush better and more frequently. Clean between your teeth with floss and interdental brushes. You need to see your own hygienist or dentist straight away for us to remove the hard, fixed tartar (calculus). This is the yellow, hard deposit that starts building up on your teeth at the gum line. Have regular scale and polishes, and listen to their top tips. Let your dental professional coach you to perfection. They can easily see where you are missing when you are cleaning, and can show you better ways. Then generally gingivitis will easily resolve and your gums return to normal.

My best advice is: get professional help to treat bleeding gums immediately!

On a personal note, I see Jennie, my hygienist, at least every 6 months and much more often if I'm run down or feeling hormonal, as this affects my gums more. You see, if I keep missing cleaning an area, and plaque sits there for over 24-48 hours, it turns into hard tartar. I can't clean that or staining away without professional help. The rough surfaces collect more and more plaque, making it impossible to keep my teeth spotless and clean.

I have to admit; I look forward to my appointments with Jennie. She is my 'Cleaning Coach,' and shows me if I am missing any areas in my mouth when I am cleaning. Jennie coaches me so I can aim for 100% clean. It is a great feeling having a super fresh mouth!

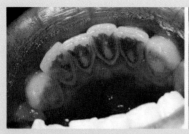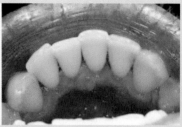

Before and after a professional scale and polish, where the tartar build-up has been removed

If gingivitis is left untreated, this can become advanced gum disease (periodontitis) and the damage is irreversible.

This is the key reason why I love visiting my hygienist. I do not want any risk of developing irreversible gum disease.

THE ADVANCED SIGNS OF GUM DISEASE

One of the signs of advanced gum disease can be detected at two metres away. The distinctive smell of bad breath is so strong. And for the person with the disease, there can be a really unpleasant taste in your mouth. This affects you and also those around you, in particular your partner.

Then the gums recede. The teeth loosen. Spaces develop between the teeth. Painful gum abscesses can occur. Finally, the teeth can simply fall out.

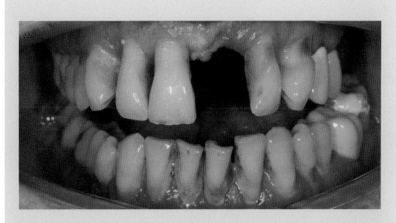

Advanced gum disease: There is severe recession of the gums with bone loss. The teeth now have spaces between them as the there is less bone support. The upper front tooth has fallen out as there is no bone left. Heavy tartar build-up is visible on the lower teeth.

WHO IS AT RISK OF GUM DISEASE?

Anyone of us who has plaque, which causes gum disease. That means everyone is at risk.

However, some people seem to be at higher risk than others. Let's take a look if you are in these high-risk groups:

- Smokers
- diabetics
- older people
- those who are malnourished with reduced nutrients
- those who are stressed
- those with a family history of gum disease
- those with a weakened immune system, for example, with HIV, diabetes or undergoing chemotherapy

CAN GUM DISEASE AFFECT OUR WHOLE HEALTH?
Now it is time to really concentrate on what you are reading!

Gum disease has serious health implications for your general health.

Gum disease is associated with an increased risk of heart disease, lung infections, diabetes and strokes.

And if affected during pregnancy, is associated with premature labour and having a baby with a low birth weight.

6 TIPS TO KEEP YOUR TEETH HEALTHY FOR LIFE

TIP 1
Reduce your intake of sugars and acids in your diet.
Keep your sugar and acid experiences to 3 times a day.
Cut down on snacking in between meals.

TIP 2
Clean your teeth perfectly twice a day, removing all
the plaque. Use a tooth brush, preferably a
rechargeable electric one. Also, clean in between your
teeth with interdental brushes and floss. Leave no
area uncleaned! Become obsessed with clean teeth, as
if you are a dentist.

TIP 3
Use a fluoride toothpaste. This hardens the enamel,
protects your teeth and can reduce decay by up to
half. Yes, you heard me correctly, half!

TIP 4
See a dentist regularly for a thorough dental
examination, perhaps every 6 months or as
recommended.

TIP 5
See a hygienist regularly and get coached in perfect
dental cleaning.

TIP 6
Never ignore bleeding gums. Ever.

TRAUMA

Sometimes we have accidents that damage our teeth, and cause teeth to be knocked out. Smiles are so beautiful. It is always so sad to see gorgeous smiles disfigured this way.

Picture this. Every Monday morning, dentists' offices across the world are filled with patients with emergencies from weekend trauma. Yet so many of these accidents are preventable!

However, there are effective steps we can all take to reduce or prevent accidents.

Breaking your teeth is irreversible. Let's take extra care!

If you have missing teeth, you already know the impact that they are having on your life.

It is time to look at the different ways to replace missing teeth. Let's look at the historical ways that have been used to replace missing teeth, but first, let's look at my top four tips for reducing tooth trauma.

4 TIPS TO REDUCE TOOTH TRAUMA

TIP 1
Wear a gum shield. Yes, you know that we should wear one for sports such as rugby and contact sports like karate. But how many teeth come out in football matches when players knock into each other? I know it's not always common or perhaps fashionable to wear one, but there are so many teeth getting knocked out through 'non-contact' sports. Let me tell you, it is really cool to have all your own teeth for life!

TIP 2
Wear a full-face helmet for mountain biking. My friend had a beautiful set of teeth until he fell off his mountain bike one day. If he had had a full-face helmet on, then his front tooth would not have met the rock. Wear a full-face helmet even when riding slow.

TIP 3
Don't walk with your hands in your pockets. How many teeth have been knocked out by simply tripping up and not having your hands ready to break your fall - teeth get knocked out!

TIP 4
Don't drink straight from a glass bottle. If you are about to take a drink and someone knocks you, then the glass bottle could hit your teeth. Your teeth would take the full impact and fracture. Use a straw.

"We need a solution that will get us back to eating, chewing and laughing again, replacing our missing teeth for the long-term."

REPLACING TEETH HISTORICALLY

THE REALITY OF DENTURES

Let's talk about dentures. Here are the facts. A denture is a prothesis. Acrylic false teeth are fixed into an acrylic or metal framework, sometimes known as a 'plate'. This is held in place with clasps or by friction alone.

In the case of a full denture, then the denture rests on the gums with a little suction from saliva or with the use of denture adhesive.

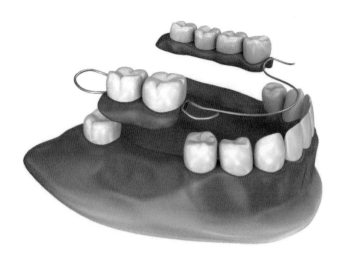

Partial denture replacing several back teeth with metal clasps to help retention

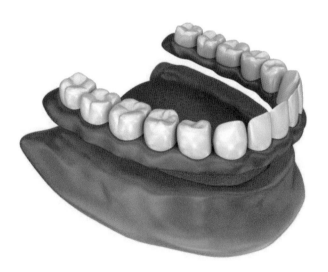

Full denture replacing all the teeth, resting on the gums.

What do they feel like?

Imagine having your arm amputated and a prosthetic arm fitted. Imagine having to learn how to use your new arm, taking it off at night, showering and bathing without it, then refitting it. Imagine not having any sensation or feelings in your prosthetic hand. Imagine the rubbing and soreness of the area where the prosthetic arm is attached to your natural skin. There are some things you will never be able to do again. Having your teeth removed and a removeable prosthesis, a denture, is similar. It is a real disability.

> "To be quite honest, dentures make people miserable, they really do. Dentures stop people from socialising. They stop them from eating everything that they like, and they can't wait to get them out. It's so sad if they have to live with these things for the rest of their lives."
>
> Jade Tichener, Practice Manager,
> Andrea Ubhi Dentistry.

With natural teeth, when we eat, we can feel the temperature of foods through our teeth and gums. We can feel texture and consistency - the crunch of crisp apples, the chewing sensation of eating steak. We can taste the foods through sensors in the roof of our mouths. We can feel the delightful resistance of chewing sticky foods.

When we have a denture, these pleasures fade.

REDUCED BITING FORCE

Imagine biting with your natural back teeth together. There is significant force applied. Up to 150-250psi in fact. Enough to chew through tough, fibrous and chewy foods.

However, dentures sit on the gums. When we bite with a denture, the force goes directly onto this soft skin. The maximum force of a full denture wearer is just 50psi, and after wearing dentures for over 15 years, the biting force can reduce to as low as 5.6psi.

This is 2% of the biting force as it used to be with healthy natural teeth.

A denture-wearer simply isn't able to bite and chew as well as when they had natural teeth.

When the dentures move and rub, ulcers can occur.

GIVING UP NUTRITIOUS FOODS

If you can't chew well, then you stop eating difficult foods. You give up the foods that you love, foods that are healthy, such as highly fibrous fruit, vegetables, nuts, seeds and maybe lean meats.

We know which healthy foods we should be eating, and the problem is that most of these require chewing.

If we can't chew our food properly and our food reaches our stomachs inadequately chewed, then we have an increased risk of stomach disorders, as partially chewed food is more difficult to digest.

"One of the things that I notice if a patient has a tooth out and they leave the space is this. All of a sudden, many develop gastrointestinal issues because they can't chew their food as well as they normally would. They just end up swallowing food half chewed. Then they get acid reflux and end up on daily medication. It's crazy, isn't it? Even just after having one tooth out."

Kate Keating, Straumann.

INCREASED RISK OF DECAY AND GUM DISEASE

Partial dentures sit next to natural teeth, and there is an increased risk of decay and gum disease unless appropriately designed and looked after, so other options may be less risky to the remaining teeth. [24]

WHY EVERY DENTURE BECOMES LOOSER IN TIME

The bone in your jaw needs a root in it to maintain its shape. Without this, over time the bone shrinks away forever.

However tight a new denture may be on the initial fitting; it will always become looser and looser over time. Every time. Because of life-long shrinkage of the bone.

We often have patients come asking for our help. Several months earlier, they have had a fabulous denture made by their dentist, and they were so happy with it initially, then all of a sudden, we hear them say, "this denture is no good" or "the denture doesn't fit". The denture hasn't changed, it's the bone supporting it that has altered.

Many patients use denture fixatives to fix their loose dentures in place. Fixatives are a gloopy, sticky gel used to temporarily stick the denture to the gums. Denture fixative can get mixed up with food and tastes disgusting, and the sensation is uncomfortable. Fixative is really difficult to remove at the end of the day. Note that fixatives are normally recommended for *once a day* application. Any further applications, may cause an overdose of ingredients such as zinc. Zinc in high doses can cause gastric irritation, headaches, irritability, lethargy, anemia and dizziness. So, if you have to use it, be cautious.

EMBARRASSMENT

Let's face it. Loose dentures are embarrassing.

A denture-wearer has to be careful how they talk, actively holding the denture in place with tongue pressure so they don't make clicking sounds and whistle through their teeth. They must be really careful when they laugh, so the denture doesn't fall out.

One patient came to our clinic. He explained that he was so embarrassed. His small grandson kept asking him to do "the trick." Once when they had both been playing together and laughing, this gentleman's denture had flown out and the grandson had never forgotten grandad's 'trick.'

Life can be tough.

IMPACTING LOVE LIFE

Dentures must be taken out at night and soaked overnight in a disinfection solution - every night. This prevents fungal infections in the mouth.

I am not going to say any more how this can affect life in the bedroom.

DETERIORATING FACIAL AESTHETICS

Denture teeth can rarely be placed in a really good aesthetic position that supports the lips and cheeks fully, and this is why.

When full dentures are made, the dentist takes impressions of the gums in the mouth and records the average positions of the moving muscles of the tongue and cheeks.

The dentures are then made to sit in the position of *minimum muscle movement*, with the tongue pushing the denture from the inside and the lips and cheeks from the outside. This is called the **neutral zone**. In this position the denture has the least chance of being kicked out of position by these muscles, and has the highest chance of stability.

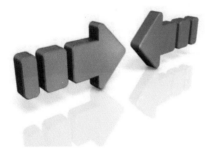

However, the problem with this is that the most aesthetic position for your teeth is somewhere much further out in a position that will give maximum support for your lips and cheeks, giving your face fullness where the bone has shrunk away. If denture teeth were placed in the position of maximum aesthetics, then the muscles of the lips and cheeks would put so much pressure on the denture, that the denture would be pushed inwards and be highly unstable.

Dentures have many draw-backs. We normally use dentures in our clinic as a temporary measure in certain cases, just for a few weeks or months while healing is occurring before permanent treatment can be provided.

The second traditional option for replacing missing teeth is a dental bridge. These have been very popular. Let's take a look and see how they compare.

THE MATTER OF DENTAL BRIDGES

Another option for replacing missing teeth is the dental bridge. This is possible if there are natural teeth next to the space.

Let me explain the procedure where one tooth is missing:

1. After extraction of a failed tooth, healing is allowed for as long as possible, so as much of the immediate bone loss can occur, typically 3 months or so.

2. Then the adjacent natural teeth are ground down on all sides by approximately 2-3 mm.

3. The bridge is then constructed in a lab by a ceramist. The bridge spans the gap with 3 teeth fixed together and is then fitted, being bonded in place.

Take a look at the following diagrams.

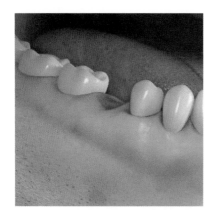

A missing tooth.

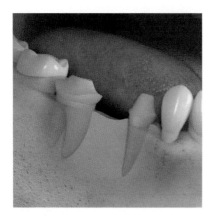

The two teeth either side of the space are ground down ready to receive the bridge.

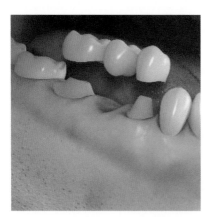

The 3-unit bridge is fitted and bonded in place permanently.

This procedure takes about 1-3 weeks, allowing time for the lab to construct the bridge, during which time a temporary bridge would normally be placed.

So, two teeth are now doing the work of 3 teeth.

However, there is another problem with this treatment.

Yes, there is significant damage to the adjacent teeth when they are ground down.

In fact, startling research shows that within 10 years, the nerve dies in approximately 30% of these living, natural teeth supporting the bridge.[25]

When the nerve of a tooth dies, this can cause pain and can cause abscess formation. The tooth may need root canal treatment.

However, listen to this.

Root canal treatment weakens the tooth structure. And it is inadvisable for a bridge to be supported by a root filled tooth as the root of the root canal treated tooth is more likely to fracture. So, if the tooth was root filled tooth prior to the making of a bridge, many dentists would decline going ahead with treatment, considering the root-filled tooth not to be strong enough to support the bridge long-term.

If you have a bridge and then you need a root canal on one of the supporting teeth, then you will find yourself between a 'rock and a hard place,' as the saying goes.

So now what do you do? You have a bridge that shouldn't be supported on a weakened tooth. Do you bite carefully for the rest of your life hoping the tooth won't fracture and the bridge fail? Do you have the bridge out and have a new longer span bridge on more healthy teeth? Or do you need to consider alternative solutions?

Another problem with a bridge is that where the tooth was lost, the remaining bone continues to shrink back indefinitely. So, at the time of fitting your new bridge, the false teeth would be snug on the gum, however over time, a gap starts to appear under it. This compromises the aesthetics, traps food and can also create spitting or whistling when speaking.

The tooth in the centre of this photo is part of a bridge, replacing a missing canine.

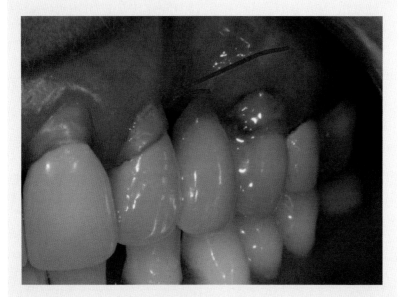

The bridge was placed years ago and would have fit perfectly up to the gum. Can you see that after many years, the bone has shrunk away, leaving a hollow in the gum/bone, where the arrow is pointing? This leaves a large space between the bridge and gum. The adjacent supporting bridge units have been repaired poorly, attempting to mask the recession.

Now bridges are tricky to clean around. A special type of floss is used to clean under the bridge area which can be fiddly. This floss has a thick harder end that is threaded under the bridge. If a bridge cannot be cleaned properly, then decay and gum disease can occur in the areas of plaque build-up.

Now, it is generally accepted among dentists that dental bridges last approx. 10 years before they fail. Then what? Well, it depends on the reason for failure.

If the supporting teeth have failed and need extracting, then the span that was one missing tooth becomes 2 or 3 missing teeth. So, the new bridge becomes larger than the last. Then the two teeth supporting the new bridge are taking even more load, and statistically, longer the span, the shorter the longevity. [26]

And when they fail, is it actually possible to make a larger bridge? Possibly not.

Why are dental bridges still being placed?

I think that the answer is this. They are just so easy in the *short-term*. They are easy for both for the patient and dentist. In just over a week or two, you can have your tooth replaced and at first, they look great. However, this is a *short-term view*.

What we need is a *life-long view.* We need a solution that will get us back to eating, chewing and laughing again, replacing our missing teeth for the long-term. Life-long.

So, what is the ideal way to replace missing teeth? What do we need in a solution?

We need a treatment that replaces missing teeth with fixed, permanent teeth. A solution that has no damage or impact to the remaining teeth and the mouth.

We need to maintain the bone level and the facial structure, gracefully supporting the skin.

We need a result that is effective, reliable and has a very high long-term success rate. A solution that is safe and has decades of solid scientific research backing it.

We need an impressive solution where the teeth feel like real teeth, function like real teeth and look like real teeth.

We need a treatment that will be so effective that it will restore our broken confidence, so we can bite, chew and laugh like we used to with a natural-feeling, healthy smile.

And we need a solution that gives the best long-term value for money.

It is time to look at dental implants.

Are you ready?

SECTION 2

DENTAL IMPLANTS, THE STATE-OF-THE-ART SOLUTION

"I was so ashamed of how my teeth used to be. Implants have given me a second chance of having a good smile."

CHRIS BROOKES

WHAT IS A DENTAL IMPLANT?

First, a very short history lesson which may surprise you.

In 1931, during a Honduran archaeological dig, a large part of a woman's jaw was found, dating back to 600AD. In that jaw, there were three teeth missing, and in their place, three tooth-shaped pieces of shell had been inserted. It wasn't until later, in 1970, when Professor Amadeo Bobbio, in Brazil, examined this same jaw with X-rays. What he found was very interesting. New bone had formed around the shells, proving that these shells had been placed while the woman was alive and that the body had 'accepted' them.

In more recent times, dental implants have been tested in the material, titanium. These have been researched and placed in humans since 1965, originally by a surgeon called Branemark. There is now over 50 years research into modern dental implants.

"A dental implant is an artificial tooth root that works like a natural one"

Sounds perfect, yet are they perfect for you?

Let's get back to the original question.

What exactly is a dental implant?

> "A dental implant is a very small but strong post made of biocompatible metals or ceramics, which is inserted into the jaw bone in place of the missing tooth root. Such an implant acts as a support for the tooth, and is surgically inserted under local anaesthetic on an outpatient basis. Until the implant is securely attached to the jaw bone (the process is called "osseointegration"), a healing phase of between 6 weeks and a few months is necessary, depending on the individual medical situation. Once healed, the artificial root acts as a base for fixing individual crowns and multi-tooth bridges. Also, the implant can be used as an anchor for entire dental prostheses."
>
> Straumann

Technically, a dental implant is made up of three parts, the *fixture*, the *abutment* and the *restoration*. I'm going to explain these three words, and I want you to remember them, as they will come up again. Let me explain.

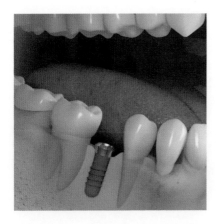

The implant fixture only.

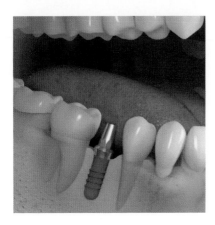

The fixture with the abutment in place.

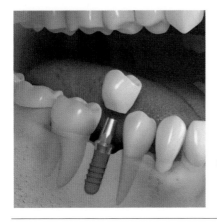

The fixture with abutment and crown.

THE FIRST PART: THE IMPLANT FIXTURE

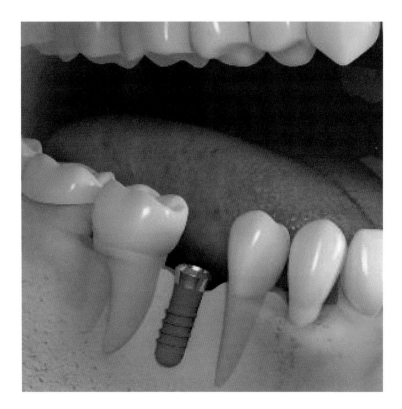

The fixture replaces the root of the tooth.

This is the *screw* that is gently placed into the jaw bone. I say *gently* because the procedure is provided under local anaesthetic, sometimes with sedation. Some patients say that a simple implant placement feels similar to having a filling done.

The fixture lies under the gum, normally out of sight.

Here is the technical part. There are different materials that the fixture can be made from, the main ones being titanium, ceramic and Roxolid®.

Titanium

Pure titanium is a biocompatible metal, which means that it is non-toxic and well-tolerated by the body. It is both strong and light. This is why it has been used for so many medical uses, like

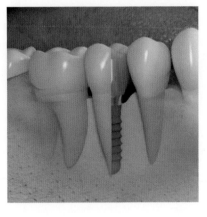

surgical implements and joint replacements.

Titanium has a high strength and low weight. One of its most important medical applications is in implants, and those made from titanium have been shown to bond very well to living bone. This bonding process by the body is called

osseointegration. Because of this, dental implants can last for decades and for life.

Ceramic

Ceramic implants are made from an ivory-coloured, zirconia ceramic. However, these are not as popular yet, as the advantages of titanium and Roxolid appear to outweigh

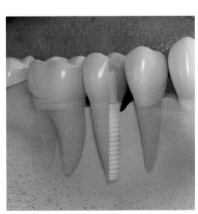

ceramic. Ceramic is a great solution for those patients with an allergy to titanium.

Roxolid®

Roxolid® is a titanium-zirconium alloy which is stronger than pure titanium and has excellent osseointegration properties.

Roxolid is unique to one manufacturer, and this is one of the reasons that we use the

Straumann dental implant system, because by combining the biocompatibility of the titanium with the strength of the Zirconia, there is a stronger material than just titanium.

This means that smaller fixtures can be placed which are just as strong, perhaps avoiding the need of bone grafting where there is reduced bone. This in turn reduces the overall cost and speeds up treatment time. Roxolid® shows faster healing and higher treatment predictability.

> "Roxolid, means that now we can use much smaller implants. So, implants are more easily placed in patients who have reduced bone. We see this problem affecting older patients often. Perhaps they could not have had implants 10 years ago, now, that's not necessarily the case. Now they can have simple implant procedures with these more modern, smaller yet stronger implant fixtures. These patients are actually able to have treatment that can significantly increase their quality of life."
>
> Kate Keating, Straumann.

Advances in the Surface Technology of Implant Fixtures

Research has been done to see if the healing time and predictability can be improved by different surfaces on dental implant fixtures. A new advance has come in the form of Straumann SLActive® which is clinically proven to shorten the healing time and can increase treatment predictability.

Advances are coming all the time. Dental implantology is a major growth area. However, as with all advances in science, progress lies in solid research proving success over time.

THE SECOND PART: THE ABUTMENT

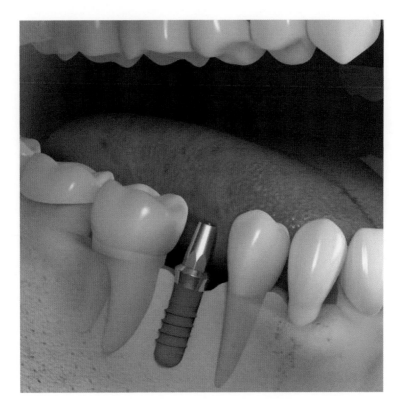

The implant fixture is hollow at the top with an internal screw-like surface. Remember Meccano when you were a kid, where one section attaches to the next and then another to that one?

The abutment is screwed into the fixture. This is the substructure, ready to take the visible restoration. The main reason that this is not normally already integrated into the fixture, is that the abutment can be made up of different shapes, depending on the design of the *restoration* which fixes onto the abutment. The restoration can be so varied in design, that there needs to be different shapes of the abutment to create the best aesthetics at the end.

THE THIRD PART: THE RESTORATION

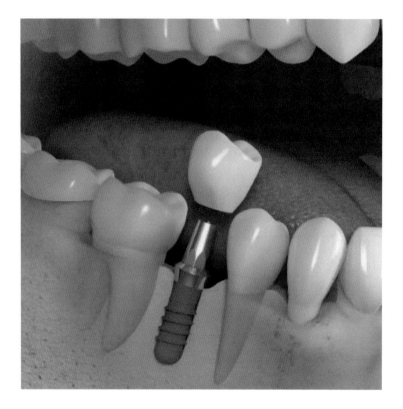

This is the section you see above the gum is the *restoration*.

There are several ways of restoring an implant, depending on how many teeth are missing, including a single crown replacing a single tooth, a dental bridge on several implants replacing several or all the missing teeth or a denture which is fixed in place with implants.

Let's talk about these in more detail.

REPLACING A SINGLE MISSING TOOTH

If there is a single tooth missing, then you will need a single implant with a single crown on the abutment and fixture. The crown is placed securely and will remain in place like a natural tooth.

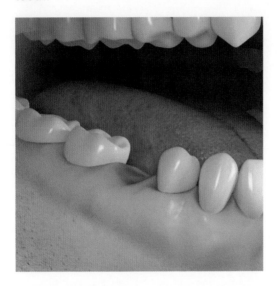

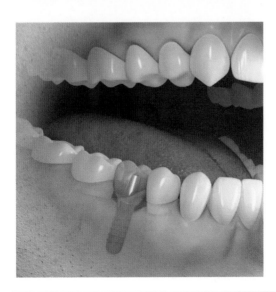

REAL EXAMPLE

REPLACING A FRACTURED TOOTH WITH A DENTAL IMPLANT

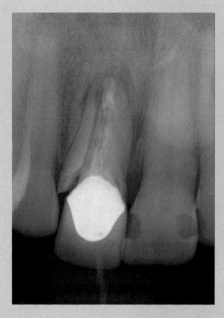

CASE 1 X-RAY: before

This patient's natural tooth had a fractured root after the tooth, after being previously root-filled and crowned (the white is the metal substructure of the crown).

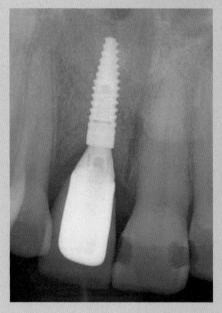

CASE 1 X-RAY: after

The failed tooth has been removed and replaced with the implant fixture, abutment and crown.

Case by Dr Adam Glassford.

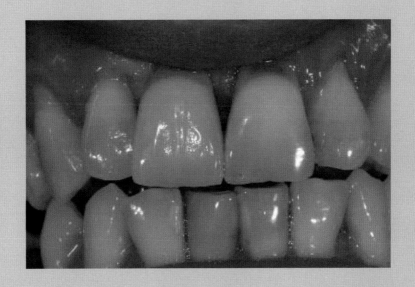

CASE 1 Photo: after

The final implant crown made to match the existing teeth.

Case by Dr Adam Glassford.

REPLACING SEVERAL MISSING TEETH

If there are several missing teeth, then multiple implant fixtures are placed, and an implant-bridge is fitted permanently on top of them. This bridge is fixed securely.

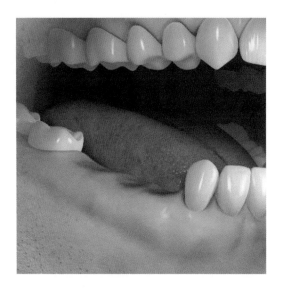

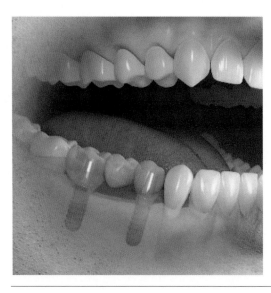

Note: an *implant-retained bridge* is not to be confused with a *tooth-retained bridge*. In both cases a *bridge* is used, however the *implant-retained bridge* has the bridge attached to implants rather than teeth.

REAL EXAMPLE

Replacing Several Upper Front Teeth with Dental Implants

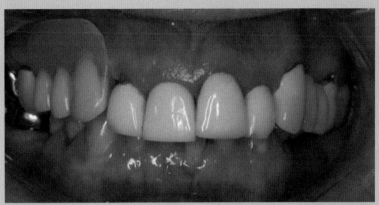

CASE 2: Before

Several back teeth were missing and had been replaced with a partial denture which had become loose and ill-fitting (see the left side of the photo), the remaining teeth had failing crowns and bridges with recession.

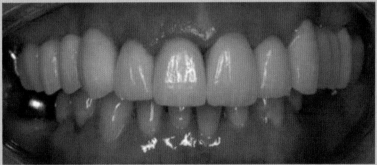

CASE 2: After

An implant-retained bridge replaced the loose partial denture, and the remaining upper teeth were restored with new crowns. Case by Dr Adam Glassford.

REPLACING A FULL JAW OF MISSING TEETH

If all the teeth are missing in your jaw then there are three implant-based solutions:

OPTION 1: IMPLANT-RETAINED FIXED BRIDGE

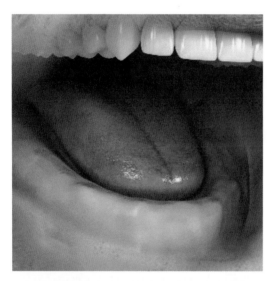

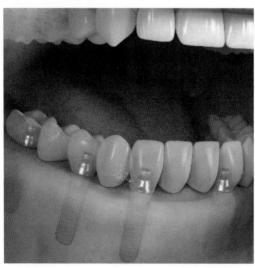

This is the ideal option if you would like fixed-in teeth.

 At our clinic, this is the most popular choice for those missing all of their teeth.

Why? Because the teeth are fixed permanently in place. They look like teeth. When you bite, you can bite fully.

Apples and steak are easy.

Four to eight implants are placed into the jaw. The number of implants used depends on several factors, including bone levels and risk factors. Then a dental bridge is made to carry the new teeth. The implant-bridge uniquely fits the jaw, mouth and facial shape. The implant-bridge is secured in place and not removed, so it will be cleaned in situ with a tooth brush and interdental cleaning brushes and floss.

This is the next best thing to having your own natural teeth. The look of the teeth and the aesthetics can be made specifically to suit your face-shape as the teeth can be placed in the best position to support your overlying skin. The restoration does not need to be in the compromised *neutral zone* as a full denture does as this restoration is precision fitted to the implant fixtures which are solidly integrated into the jaw bone.

They look natural and the bite functions normally. You should be able to eat everything like you used to with natural teeth.

However, this option is the trickiest to clean around. You will need to master interdental brushes and floss.

If there is a question of your ability to clean around your new implants, then the removeable option next may be a better option, so your implants stay healthy for life.

REAL EXAMPLE

REPLACING FAILING UPPER TEETH WITH FULL JAW IMPLANTS

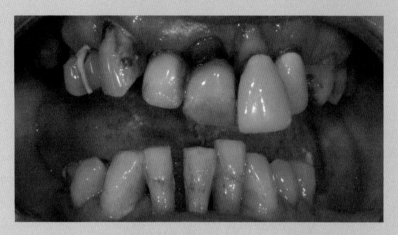

CASE 3: before

All the upper the teeth are failing.

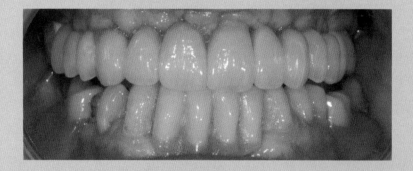

CASE 3: after

The upper teeth have been replaced with an Implant-Retained Fixed Bridge. Case by Dr Adam Glassford.

OPTION 2: DENTURE STABILISATION ON IMPLANT-LOCATORS

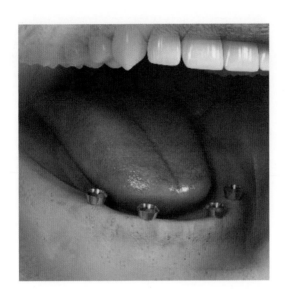

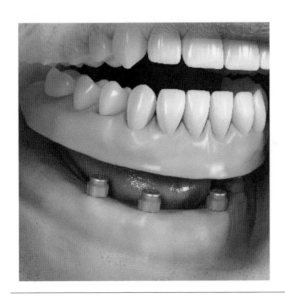

This is a simple solution for loose dentures by simply clipping the denture onto implants like press-studs. Two to four implant fixtures are inserted into the lower jaw and a minimum of four in the upper jaw. Again, the number of implants used depends on many factors, including bone quality, risk factors and cost. The press-stud attachments on the implants have opposing attachments within the denture. This allows the denture to be pressed into the mouth and 'clicked' into place. Although there can be slight movement with this type of removeable restoration, it is a world away from an unsecured complete denture and offers security, stability and confidence.

A major drawback of this option is that the denture is required to be removed several times a day for cleaning and kept out at night for disinfection.

This option is the cheapest full jaw solution.

Your ability to eat and chew will significantly increase with this option, however if you want to really bite into apples and crusty bread, then you might want to consider the Implant-Retained Fixed Bridge.

REAL EXAMPLE

UPPER AND LOWER - DENTURE STABILISATION ON IMPLANT-LOCATORS

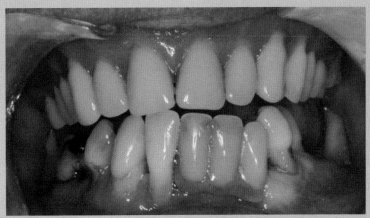

CASE 4: before

This patient had a full denture replacing the missing teeth in the upper jaw, and a partial denture on the lowers with some failing remaining teeth.

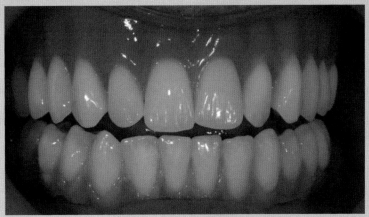

CASE 4: after
Upper and lower jaws were restored with full dentures on Implant-Locators. Case by Dr Adam Glassford.

OPTION 3: DENTURE STABILISATION ON AN IMPLANT-RETAINED BAR

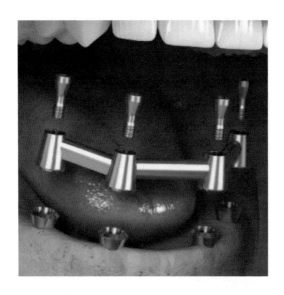

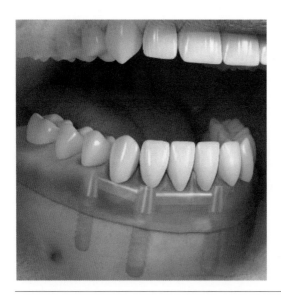

This option is a step up from option 2 and suits the patient who is looking for a much more secure removeable option. And in particular, in the upper jaw, if you are tired of your denture covering the roof of your mouth, preventing you tasting and feeling foods, then with this option, your denture base can be really small, allowing the roof of the mouth to remain uncovered.

In the upper jaw, this generally requires placement of four implants per jaw. A custom-made bar is fitted which allows a minimal denture to be secured using clips and studs. This denture has a metal base and can be much smaller and more discreet than a regular denture, while still providing great aesthetics.

This is a very rigid and robust solution, and you should be able to eat apples and crusty bread using this type of solution. This option has significant stability advantages over the implant-locator style attachment, as the bar-retained denture has increased rigidity.

Again, a drawback of this option is that the denture is required to be removed twice daily for cleaning, and is kept out overnight for disinfection.

HOW SUCCESSFUL ARE DENTAL IMPLANTS?

Success depends on whether the body accepts the dental implant fixture and bonds with it.

Research by Straumann, one of the largest worldwide implant manufacturers, whose clinicians have placed over 14 million of their implants, suggests that success occurs in 98% of implants. We have a slightly higher success rate than that at 98.9%.

> "If an implant fixture fails to integrate with the bone, we will be able to spot this on an x-ray before the final restoration is fitted on top. If this happens, the implant is simply removed and then replaced after a few weeks of healing. There is normally no pain associated with this. The fixture may simply become loose. In general, failure is due to poor healing such as in the case of diabetics and heavy smokers, however it can occur for unknown reasons in healthy individuals. Failure rates are so low, that most surgeons would provide a replacement implant at no additional cost,"
>
> Dr Adam Glassford.

Success depends on several things, including:

- The health of the patient

- If the patient is a smoker

- The quality of the implant placed

- The position the implant is placed in

- Appropriate loading of the implant

- The skill of the surgeon who places it

- The quality of the aftercare

- How well the implant is cared for by the patient.

We are going to discuss this in much more detail later, but first. Listen to this.

HOW ARE BITING FORCES AFFECTED AFTER IMPLANTS?

The biting force of natural teeth is about 150-250 psi. With full dentures, this can drop to 5.6 psi. With dental implants, our biting and chewing ability returns to normal, in fact higher than with natural teeth, reaching up to 300+psi on average. So why are the forces achieved with implants be so high? Implant fixtures are fitted directly into the bone, whereas teeth have a ligament which acts as a cushion for the tooth.

LET'S SUMMARISE

- **Dental implants merge with our body.**

  Even the best prosthesis will always be a foreign part. By contrast, a dental implant is simply an artificial root. When cared for, dental implants are expected to last a lifetime.

- **Dental implants give secure confidence to talk and laugh.**

  Dental implants are fixed securely in place, eliminating the worry that a denture will fall out.

- **No more embarrassment of smiling with missing teeth.**

- **Life can become more fulfilled.**

  We become more engaging to be around and studies show we appear more appealing.

  We can be comfortable around our nearest and dearest, day and night, as we know we will keep our teeth firmly fixed in place.

  Our career prospects can flourish as we regain our confidence as our smiles are beautiful and bright.

- **Dental implants increase the chances of keeping our remaining teeth healthy.** The bone stays strong and the adjacent teeth are kept whole and healthy without any bridge preparation of adjacent healthy teeth.

- **Bone volume remains intact.**

Our face height stays normal and the bone volume supporting our cheeks remains, minimising premature aging by maintaining the structure under the skin on our face and lips.

☑ **With dental implants, biting and chewing ability returns to normal.**

In fact, chewing forces become even stronger than natural teeth, providing the forces that we need to eat the healthy and nutritious foods that we love. The biting force with natural teeth is 150-250 psi. With full dentures, this can drop to 5.6 psi. With dental implants, this increases to 300+psi on average.

This gives us the opportunity to keep our bodies nourished and healthy into old age.

☑ **According to the National Institute of Health, on average, we live 9.8 years longer with fixed or natural teeth than those with partial or full dentures.**

☑ **Dental implants preserve the facial structure, keeping us looking younger.**

Implants transmit chewing forces to the jaw bone. This is not the case if teeth are missing or when a conventional prosthesis has been put in place. If these forces cease, the bone may slowly recede and the shape of the face may change over time.

"The brave man
is not he who
does not feel
afraid, but he
who conquers
that fear."

NELSON MANDELA

DEALING WITH FEAR

However, before we go any further, let's deal with the problem of fear. If you get sweaty palms when thinking of the dentist, then you are definitely not alone.

In fact, you are probably struggling to concentrate on reading this book at this point and you may already have increased heart rate just thinking about surgery.

Many people are scared of the dentist and this is one of the key reasons why they have allowed their teeth and gums to deteriorate.

We understand. We fully understand.

Some people may have had a bad experience with an unsympathetic dentist. However, picture this.

There are many, many of us dentists who love our patients and live for our profession. We feel blessed, quite frankly, that we have been given the opportunity to help our patients get their smiles back. Our ultimate moments are when we help our patients move forwards with healthy, happy smiles that last a life-time. There are many, many dentists like this. So, find a dentist that you really like and who puts you at your ease. Keep looking until you find your 'forever-dentist' who suits you perfectly.

I know that some of you are desperate to have dental implants, however, you simply feel that the surgical procedure is beyond you. Well there is an amazing solution to this.

Here is the magic word.

SEDATION

Sedation is a way of having all your treatment without the anxiety. With sedation, you will be conscious and awake, however you will feel so relaxed that you will not be bothered about what is going on around you.

Sedation has an amnesiac effect too, so you will forget about the procedure too. Fantastic!

Sedation makes treatment easy and possible.

At our clinic, we suggest that patients have sedation for all implant placements. It makes the procedure an easy and lovely experience. However, some patients prefer not to, and that's ok too.

Intravenous sedation is a way that we can remove the anxiety surrounding a dental treatment. We often use this with anxious or phobic patients for any dental procedure, and also for patients that are not normally anxious but are having certain treatments such as bone grafting or multiple implants.

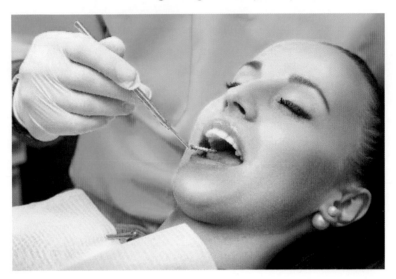

THE BENEFITS

- total removal of anxiety from the moment it is given
- amnesia, so you will not remember the procedure
- no 'hangover' afterwards
- a feeling of relaxation for the rest of the day and night
- reduction in any bruising or swelling, due to the effect of the sedative safely lowering your blood pressure

HOW IT IS DONE?

The sedative is given via a small cannula is placed in the back of the hand.

How Safe is Sedation?

"I have carried out over 2000 IV sedations over the past 22 years and I train other dentists in this valuable technique. I believe that dental IV sedation is extremely safe and there has never been a death in the UK with this technique. IV sedation has now mainly replaced general anaesthetics in dentistry due to its safety statistics,"

Dr Adam Glassford.

Before Your Sedation Appointment

Your medical history will be checked to ensure that any medication or medical conditions that you have do not interfere with the sedative. It is important to provide full and accurate information about ANY medicine, drug, tablet or treatment that you are currently receiving. It is also important to inform us about any sedative that you have been on recently and any alcohol intake.

You can eat and drink as normal before sedation but I advise that you do not have a large meal 2 hours of less, prior to sedation. The 'nil by mouth' concept relates to hospital general anaesthetics and NOT to sedation so please do not starve yourself! You should eat normally and take all medication normally on the day of your appointment. It is important that you do not drink any alcohol on the evening of the sedation as it may have a stronger effect than normal.

During Your Visit

It is best to wear flat shoes as you may be unsteady on your feet immediately after the sedation. Please wear loose-sleeved clothing as we will need to use a vein in your hand or arm. Any nail varnish should be removed from 2 fingers on each hand, so we can place a monitoring device on your finger. This shines a light through your finger tip to monitor your pulse and oxygen. Clear nail varnish is fine and does not need removing.

It is extremely important that you have a responsible adult escort that will take you home afterwards. You will NOT be able to drive a car for 24 hours, so please bear this in mind when planning your appointment. You must avoid performing any dangerous tasks for 24 hours following sedation as your co-ordination may be affected.

"It was completely different to what I had thought."

CHRISTINE

THE IMPLANT JOURNEY STEP BY STEP

Let's talk in detail about what can you expect during your dental implant journey.

THE CONSULTATION

Your consultation is the key time to find out what treatment is appropriate for you, what your options are and to learn about your surgeon.

At your consultation, your surgeon will need to learn your medical history to make sure there is nothing there that will contraindicate treatment.

The surgeon will also ask you how much you drink or smoke. I know you really want implants, but you must be honest as the success of treatment depends on it. My advice, don't lie and waste your money!

You will be asked what your concerns are, and whether you have any other thoughts about your smile that might influence treatment. For example, if you have been thinking of having whiter teeth, then that needs discussing and making part of your treatment plan from the beginning. We don't want a beautiful new implant crown matching your natural yellow teeth perfectly if you don't want yellow teeth!

All the options and pros and cons will be discussed with you. It is the surgeon's responsibility to cover all bases.

THE CBCT SCAN

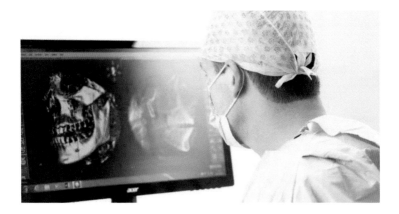

CBCT means 'Cone Beam Computed Tomography' and is more commonly known as a 'CT scan.' This is a 3-dimensional x-ray. It shows the width of the bone and the height. It also shows where your nerves, arteries and veins are situated.

The positioning of your implant and grafting can be planned extremely accurately and safely, to fractions of a millimetre, to allow precise, safe surgery.

Standard x-rays of your remaining teeth may also be taken to screen for gum disease and decay, which will normally be treated first.

THE TREATMENT PLAN

Your surgeon will give you a written treatment plan. This will describe all the treatment options, which treatment is considered to be the most appropriate for you and all the associated costs.

The information will include all the risks and benefits.

It will also discuss the option of sedation.

Normally this is a lengthy document, so make yourself a cup of tea and take the time to read it thoroughly.

You may have additional questions, so you must get these answered to be able to make an informed decision. You will be able to call the surgeon's Treatment Coordinator or arrange a second consultation with the surgeon for further discussion.

"Will I be without teeth at any stage?"

This is an important question we get asked all the time. A temporary restoration such as a denture or immediate loaded crown or bridge can be made during the healing stages until you are ready to have the permanent restoration fitted. Check with your surgeon before you begin.

THE TREATMENT STAGES

STEP 1: BONE GRAFTING

Not everyone needs bone grafting, however, if you have had significant bone loss, you may need a little more bone and this problem can be solved with a bone graft. We are going to discuss this in much more detail later.

Bone grafting gets the site ready for the implant fixtures, and often the graft is left to heal for 3-9 months before the next stage.

STEP 2: IMPLANT FIXTURE PLACEMENT

The implant placement is a surgical procedure carried out under local anaesthesia and often under sedation.

We access the site by numbing the area fully and make a cut in the gum. Then we use some small drills to create a hole for the implant, then place the implant into this hole. After we have placed the implant, your gum will be closed level to the gum either side using a 'healing abutment.'

If there is a defect in the bone that will need filling in at the time of implant placement, and a material to build out the bone volume may be placed. Painkillers and antibiotics may be prescribed for 1 week following the procedure to help minimise the chance of infection.

In general, a single implant placement is associated with minimal pain and discomfort afterwards. During the procedure itself you will not experience any pain at all, as we use a very effective local anaesthetic to numb the area being worked on.

Most patients report that over-the-counter pain killers are needed for the day of treatment but generally there is little or no pain the day after.

Immediate Post-Operative Care

Plan the implant placement so that you are not going on holiday or have any special occasions immediately afterwards in case you have some swelling or bruising visible. Plan to eat soft foods for 3-4 days afterwards to ensure that the stitches are not disturbed during the very important initial healing time. Foods such as fish, soups, mashed potato are ideal. Avoid crusty breads and hard chewy foods during this time. Avoid alcohol and aspirin for 24 hours afterwards as this can lead to additional bleeding or bruising.

Depending on the individual case, an immediate temporary restoration may be placed on the implant during the healing stage. This allows you to enjoy a natural looking smile quite early in the process. If a temporary immediate crown has been fitted, it is very important that you eat softer foods on this for the first 4 weeks following treatment to ensure the implant is not disturbed during healing.

"Some people walk out as if they've not had anything done. Twice this week, we had it when patients just walked out after implant surgery and went and did their shopping. A lot of patients are anxious about what is involved and really, it's easy.

It is different if patients have had extensive bone grafting. They are going to want to go home and put their feet up for a few days. "

Jade Tichener,
Assistant Practice Manager at Andrea Ubhi Dentistry

Removal of Stitches

This is carried out 7-14 days after surgery and only takes a few minutes. In general, there is no need for local anaesthetic during suture removal as it is a quick and simple procedure.

STEP 3: THE HEALING PHASE

The implant is given time to bond with your bone, otherwise known as *osseointegration*. This normally takes between 3 weeks and a few months. This depends on the individual medical situation, the quality of your existing bone and the type of surface the implant has.

The healing time can be reduced by using implants with SLActive®surface (Straumann), normally reducing healing to 2-3 weeks.

STEP 4: THE RESTORING PHASE

Exposure of the Implant Fixture

After a period of around 3-4 months, your implant will be ready to restore. However, it may initially need to be *exposed,* if your gum has healed over the top of it. This is a simple procedure done under local anaesthetic where a small cut is made in the gum over the implant and an elongated metal cylinder called a *healing abutment* is screwed onto the implant and allowed to protrude slightly out of the gum. Your gum will then heal around this. The procedure usually only takes 15-30 minutes and there is usually no discomfort afterwards.

In many cases, this stage can be bypassed by fitting the healing abutment at the time of implant placement as long as the bone if solid enough to allow this.

Impression of the Fixture

The final impression is taken around 10-12 weeks after the implant has been placed. This is a very simple procedure, which can usually be done without any local anaesthetic. The impressions are very similar to those done when a crown is being made for a natural tooth. This appointment takes around 30 minutes in the case of a single implant.

The shade of your new teeth is taken at this appointment, being matched to your remaining teeth. If you want whiter teeth, then you may need to have started professional teeth whitening before this stage, so we can match to the new shade of your remaining natural teeth. If all your teeth are being replaced, then the colour is simply decided by you.

These records are sent to the laboratory.

Your personalised new teeth are created at the dental lab.

Placement of the Final Restoration

Once the lab has custom-made your personal restoration, that is unique to you, this final restoration is tried-in and then fitted, being connected securely to the implant fixtures. The bite is carefully checked so that the teeth meet evenly. You will be carefully shown how to clean around your new restoration.

This is an overview of the treatment process. Each case will need to be individually tailored to suit each unique situation.

STEP 5: HYGIENE COACHING

At a return visit a week or two later, your surgeon will check your restoration and in particular, double check the bite, so that you are comfortable and functioning normally.

Your hygienist will check how you are cleaning, and give you coaching for oral hygiene. This is the most important part of treatment. Why? Because the next stage of success depends on you!

When I was writing this book, I asked some of our team their thoughts about working with dental implants. Two of our senior nurses said this. I think it shows how much they love their jobs! In fact, I am not sure they would call it a 'job,' more of a Life=Calling.

"When I first started working with dental implants, I didn't understand the scope at all. They can replace any missing teeth, from one, two, several to full mouth replacement.
I just love watching our patients' journeys and patients being totally amazed. They become so happy and confident. It is so nice to see this. I love my job; it is so fulfilling."

Michelle Harrall

Senior Dental Nurse to Dr Adam Glassford

"It is very satisfying nursing for the Implantologist as it requires meticulous planning to the highest standards to ensure optimum results for each patient. The results are amazing and it's great to see the reactions from our patients at the end of their treatments."

Kim Littlefair

Senior Dental Nurse at Andrea Ubhi Dentistry

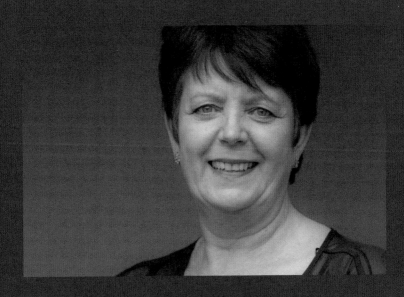

"My dentist referred me for a dental implant to be done. It was a good experience, completely different to what I had thought, less painful. I thought there would be more involved.

It was brilliant. I just had local anaesthetic. It wasn't sore at all. Absolutely straight forward. I can bite an apple now, whereas I would have never done that before as my tooth would have broken off."

CHRISTINE

"If you don't care for your implants carefully and diligently, then they will fail.

Simple as that."

AFTER CARE

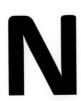**ow listen carefully, as this is the most important part of having implants.**

I cannot stress this enough.

What you will learn here makes the difference between success and failure of dental implants.

Yes, having implants is like getting your natural teeth back. Your teeth need a lot of care or they will fail, as you may have had deep personal experience of. To keep your implants healthy, there is a joint responsibility between you, and your dentist or hygienist.

However, the ultimate responsibility is yours.

Some people think that having dental implants is a 'Forget-About-Them-Afterwards' procedure. They think that if they throw money at their problem and get the best surgeon, then they have no responsibility.

Not at all.

COMMITTING TO A U-TURN
Time for some delicate honesty.

Often the key reason why you need dental implants is because of lack of care of your natural teeth. If you choose to have dental implants, then you are committing to a complete U-turn in your attitude to care of your mouth or you should not bother having this potentially life-changing treatment.

There is no point.

If you don't care for your implants carefully and diligently, then they will fail. Simple as that. If you care for them and clean them properly, then they should last a life-time.

At our clinic, if you attend for a consultation and you need help with your oral hygiene, we will not rush into implant treatment. We want your implants to be successful for life and we know that depends on your commitment to caring for them.

So, before we commit to placing implants for you, our hygienist will provide sessions to help you and coach you to clean your mouth so it is sparkling and fresh. Our hygienist, will keep coaching you and keep coaching you until you get it. We will work with you so that you can be ready for implants. Your mouth will be as healthy as possible, with harmful bacteria eliminated, so your body can accept implant treatment successfully.

You are going to love your fresh, clean, healthy mouth!

Then, and only then, will our surgeon consider placing dental implants.

We want your treatment to be 100% successful. For that to be a possibility, you need a 100% clean mouth with 100% commitment to keeping your mouth clean.

KEEPING YOUR IMPLANT HEALTHY

Implant health is mainly determined by how clean you keep your whole mouth and implant. Therefore, hygiene appointments are recommended as often as necessary after surgery, at least every 3-6 months. You will need to see a hygienist who is trained in caring for dental implants. You see, the titanium fixture can be scratched with traditional hygienist tools, so special implant-compatible ones are used.

Plaque is the soft, white film that builds up when we don't clean our teeth perfectly, often in the very difficult to reach crevices of our mouth. We know that any plaque that is left for more than 24 hours, then it turns hard, into *calculus*, also known as *tartar*.

The hygienist will clean any hard tartar away so that you can clean perfectly again. You will be coached to clean any difficult areas. Then you can clean impeccably again.

"Let me say this again. If you don't clean around your implants, then there is a high risk of failure"

This responsibility of caring for your implants is all yours, and your implant and hygiene team is there to support and help you achieve this.

At our practice, we give every patient a complimentary hygiene appointment immediately after their restorations are fitted to show you how to clean around your new implants. We demonstrate the best tools for the job - often an ultrasonic electric toothbrush, interdental brushes and floss.

ANNUAL IMPLANT CHECKS

Your surgeon or trained general dentist will provide annual implant checks for life. At this appointment, the health of the implant is checked and your remaining teeth are checked for signs of gum disease or decay.

You will have X-rays taken of the implant annually at least for the first 5 years to check the health of the implant and check for any signs of bone loss, which could require therapy.

A WORD OF WARNING

Go a little easy on your new implants when you are biting and chewing! You are going to be so excited to eat like you used to. However, even natural enamel can't cope with hard biting into pork crackling, ice cubes or fruit stones without fracturing. The implant restorations are of a similar hardness to enamel - so the ceramic restorations will also break like natural teeth if mis-used!

Remember Rob, who lost a tooth after his year in Australia? Let's hear the end to his story.

> "Having an implant was dead easy. So, so simple. Just a simple injection. The surgery appointment lasted 30 mins, maybe 40 mins tops. I took two over-the-counter pain killers because my wife forced me to! No pain. No swelling. Literally nothing. Just straight back to work.
> That was 4 years ago. I've not had any trouble. My implant tooth feels just like it did before."
>
> Rob from Ferrybridge, Yorkshire.

"After teeth have been extracted, there is a clock ticking as the bone starts shrinking away"

THE ISSUE OF LOST BONE

When teeth are removed, if there is no stimulus for the remaining bone, this bone quickly shrinks away. As dentists, we call this *resorption*.

This occurs most rapidly in the first few weeks after extraction and slowly continues indefinitely.

Dental implants require a certain depth and width of bone to be strong enough to load with a restoration that will take biting forces of up to 300+psi.

Some of the initial dental implants were very big and long, as scientists thought that the bigger an implant, the stronger it would be. These long implants needed a lot of bone, so many people who had lost bone were unable to have implants.

However modern research is showing that smaller modern implants are just as strong, in fact stronger than the older, longer ones.

The Roxolid® new generation material, a combination of Zirconia and titanium, is stronger than pure titanium. So, smaller and smaller implants, some as short as 4mm, can give the same strength, are less invasive and can be placed in patients with very little remaining bone. Also, in the unusual scenario of failure, they can be more easily removed than longer ones, and therefore more easily replaced with little bone disruption.

Size really matters.

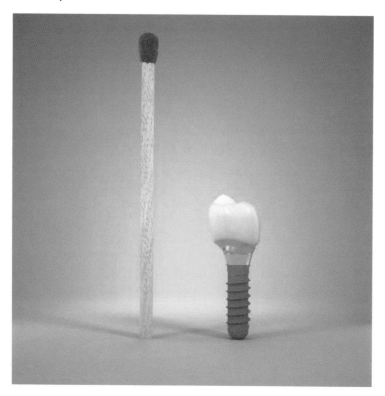

A matchstick to implant size comparison.

But what if you have lost too much bone already even for these super-small modern implants?

The answer lies in bone grafts. Now, interestingly, most patients need a certain amount of bone grafting, because they have left the site of the missing tooth long enough for the bone to have shrunk away.

Let's look at the modern world of bone grafting.

TOP TIP

If you need a tooth extracting, then plan the extraction and implant placement together with an implant surgeon BEFORE the tooth is removed. This minimizes any bone shrinkage that otherwise could occur immediately after the extraction, even in the first week or two.

The reason we are going to discuss this in detail, is that the majority of patients need bone grafting for implants, and we want you to understand that in the majority of cases, **simple** bone grafting is exactly that, a **simple** procedure.

In general, bone has the ability to regenerate completely but requires some sort of scaffold to do so. This is where bone grafts come in. They provide a scaffold for new bone to be laid down. Most bone grafts are expected to be fully reabsorbed and replaced as the natural bone heals and replaces the original graft over a few months' healing time.

WHERE DO BONE GRAFTS COME FROM?

Bone grafts can be harvested from the patient's own body, obtained from a bone bank, or are made from synthetic products, such as hydroxyapatite or other naturally occurring substances with similar mechanical properties to bone.

So, the main types of grafts are:

1. Simple: Straight-Out-The-Bottle Bone
2. More Complex:
    a. Block grafting
    b. Sinus Grafting
    c. 3D Milled Bone, such as Maxgraft bone builder

A LITTLE MORE BONE – THE SIMPLE GRAFT

Small additions of bone can be placed easily at the same time as implant fixture placement.

This artificial bone is simply taken from a bottle in the form of granules and added to the surgical site around the newly placed implant-fixture. This adds bone volume and gives strength, and also improves the aesthetics of the gums, reducing the hollowed appearance. This volume provides a little more support for your skin, lips and cheeks, improving and maintaining the aesthetics.

The mineral material used is generally a pure bone mineral derived from a bovine (cow) source. This pharmaceutical grade material has been rigorously tested over more than 20 years and is guaranteed to be free of proteins and prions to ensure safety of the product. If you have a particular objection to the use of an animal product, there is a synthetic alternative that has been available for a couple of years and appears to be as successful however the bovine source has the longest and best research behind its effectiveness.

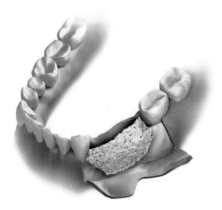

Granules of bone, simply being added at the time of surgery to add more bone volume.

MORE BONE - MORE COMPLEX GRAFTS

Sometimes there is significant bone shrinkage and resorption and a much bigger grafting procedure is necessary.

There are different techniques available including *block grafting, sinus grafting and the 3D milled MaxGraft Bonebuilder.*

Let's hear what surgeon, Dr Adam Glassford has to say.

BLOCK BONE GRAFTING
What is a block bone graft?

> When we are planning to place dental implants, if there is insufficient bone, we may need to graft a block of bone taken from elsewhere in the mouth. There are two areas that we typically take bone from: the chin area or the side of the jaw alongside the wisdom tooth. Either sites are accessed from inside the mouth. Because we are grafting your own bone, the block will fuse to the area that we place it onto and become one larger volume of bone. As the donor site heals, it refills with bone.

How do we do the block graft?

> Under sedation and local anaesthetic, a cut is made in the gum inside the mouth to access the donor and recipient sites. The block graft is carefully lifted out and then placed where it is needed, secured with small screws. The gums are sutured back. The graft is then left to heal for approximately 3 months as it fuses to the underlying bone. After healing, the screws are easily removed under local anaesthetic.

What can you expect after the graft procedure?

The graft procedure itself is painless. However, you should expect discomfort, swelling and often bruising for a few days following the graft. We will prescribe painkillers and antibiotics to minimise discomfort however you should aim to rest as much as possible for 1-7 days. We advise soft foods for a few days after the procedure.

We remove the stitches two weeks after the graft appointment and this is a very simple procedure.

What risks are associated with a block bone graft?

The graft procedure is very predictable and safe as we check the sites carefully with x-rays and CT scans beforehand as necessary. There is a very small theoretical chance of a loss of sensation to one or more of the lower teeth in the case of a chin donor site however we have not encountered such problems in the grafts we have placed. The main risks are the discomfort, swelling and bruising which should be expected afterwards.

Grafts are extremely successful but in rare cases they can fail. To date, we have not had a failure with any graft, but theoretically it can occur. Failure could be from infection or trauma to the healing area before the bone has fused. If this were to take place, the failed graft would be removed and the procedure repeated after a suitable healing time. Smokers are at a particular risk of graft failure and for this reason I do not offer block grafts in smokers. If you are a smoker but have failed to notify your surgeon of this, it is extremely important that you do so before any treatment is undertaken.

SINUS GRAFT/LIFT

In the case of the upper molar and premolar regions, a sinus lift instead of a block graft can be performed.

This procedure uses the fact that your body will lay down new bone if the membrane that lines the air sinus of the upper jaw is lifted and kept away from the natural bone for a period of time. In order to do this, under sedation and local anaesthetic, we make a hole approximately 10mm in diameter through the bone that is immediately beneath the gum next to the teeth in the upper jaw.

Once we have created this 'window,' we carefully lift the membrane of the sinus and insert a mineral material that fills the space that is created. The window is then closed over and the site allowed to heal over a period of 6-9 months.

In some cases, the sinus graft can be carried out at the same time as the implant placement. This requires around 4mm of bone to be present already. If the sinus graft can be carried out at the same time as the implant placement, the overall healing time is reduced to 4-6 months.

You will feel no pain or discomfort during the procedure.

How successful is a sinus graft?

Sinus grafts are extremely successful and have been carried out for over 20 years. Although extremely rare, a sinus graft could fail due to infection, which is why the procedure will be postponed if a patient is unwell especially with a cold or flu. In the extremely unlikely event of a failure due to infection, the sinus graft can be removed and repeated at a later date although in our experience we have not encountered this problem.

The thickness of the sinus membrane can vary and ideally, we like fairly thick and robust membranes. In some people however the membrane is very thin and can occasionally tear when we try to lift if. If this happens the sinus graft can still be carried out as we place a membrane over the tear and carry on. In a small number of cases, the tear is too wide and we need to place a membrane and close the area up to allow a new membrane to form. If this happens, as it can in around 5% of cases, we need to wait 4 to 6 weeks then carry out the procedure again.

Are there any contraindications?

Sinus grafts cannot be carried out in people that currently smoke. If you smoke, the healing of the sinus after surgery is impaired and this may lead to infection. If you smoke, then we would advise you to stop immediately and at least 3 months prior to sinus surgery.

As the sinuses are air spaces, any surgery here can be affected during the healing phase by sudden changes in atmospheric air pressure. It is advised that you do NOT: fly, scuba dive, play wind instruments such as trumpets, blow your nose forcibly, use drinking straws or engage in vigorous exercise such as gymnastics or anything involving jumping up and down for one-month following sinus surgery. After one-month, sufficient healing will have taken place to resume normal activity.

What can you expect immediately after sinus graft surgery?

You could experience pain, swelling and discomfort for a few days. We prescribe ibuprofen and antibiotics to help deal with this but you must expect some facial swelling and possibly bruising that shows on the cheeks. You will need a few days rest at home.

Some stitches will be placed in the gum after the sinus lift and these will need removing after 7-10 days. In all cases in my experience, all swelling, discomfort and bruising has gone down after 7 days.

What risks are there from sinus graft surgery?

Sinus grafting is a tried and tested procedure that has been routinely carried out for over 25 years. There are few risks beyond the initial pain and swelling but in a very small number of cases the following can occur:

- Nose bleed after surgery. This should stop within a short time.
- Bone mineral particles in the nose. This is rare but may indicate that the sinus membrane has torn possibly from sneezing. If this occurs, see your surgeon.
- Infection of the sinus after surgery. This would feel like a typical sinus pain that occurs beyond the usual 7 days of initial healing. If your sinus appears to heal, then pain starts again, it could be due to infection. If this occurs contact your surgeon.

3D MILLED BONE

This is an exciting and significant step forward. Here is how it's done.

The 3D CT scan charts the 3-dimensional volume of the existing bone in a patient's jaw. This scan is digitally sent to the laboratory, for the MaxGraft Bonebuilder, this is in Austria. From this scan, a piece of bone is designed to perfectly fit the surface of the jaw. This is custom-made for each patient, and sent back to the surgeon. At the time of surgery, the surgeon simply places the newly designed bone onto the jaw like a jigsaw puzzle. The edges match almost perfectly, which speeds up healing time.

Yes, impressive technology and the success rates are looking very, very good.

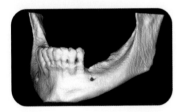 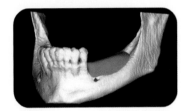

1. *the original jaw bone, showing massive bone loss where the back teeth have been lost years previously*

2. *the MaxGraft bone (in blue) in position, replacing all the missing bone, ready for dental implant placement after a healing period.*

Larger bone grafts are normally left to heal for 6 months before implant fixtures are placed.

NOTE: The amount of discomfort for all grafting procedures varies between individuals. Some people heal very quickly, and some much slower. Some people experience more pain than others. So, this is a guide based on our experience and feedback from our patients.

THE TICKING CLOCK

After teeth have been extracted, there is a clock ticking as the bone starts shrinking away.

The longer the space in the jaw is left, the more difficult it is for the surgeon to place implants and the more difficult it is for you. Surgery time is longer. Healing times are longer. The procedure becomes more expensive.

There comes a point where so much bone is lost that the even the gums have shrunk significantly. Then a surgeon simply cannot place enough grafted bone, as there is **too little gum to stretch over** any newly placed bone. Then that is when implants simply are not possible.

99% of patients who attend our clinic for consultation are suitable for dental implants. Sometimes people believe that they do not have enough bone for dental implants. However, in the hands of a surgeon experienced in advanced grafting, then solutions are possible, solid and successful: 99% of the time.

"Only after getting all the really important information, ask about price.

Only now can you compare real value."

CHOOSING A SURGEON

The most important question to ask after deciding to have implants is this. Who are you going to ask to provide your treatment?

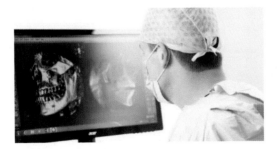

There are no dental implant qualification restrictions in the UK for dentists. Any dentist can place implants! Yes, I'm as worried as you. There are some dental implant courses that provide just a weekend introduction to dental implants and then a dentist could start placing implants!

Remember that surgeons new to placing implants, often offer loss-leading cheap fees to gain experience. So cheap may indicate a lack of experience. Note also that 'cheap' may be more expensive in the long-run, as the costs of an experienced team re-treating failed implants are much higher than providing the treatment initially.

As a profession, we would love there to be worldwide mandatory certification and for there to be mentoring programmes in place, however until we do, you, as the patient, must do your research diligently.

So, let's look at how you are going to find an experienced and competent implant surgeon.

We are going to give you as many tips and advice as we possibly can.

UNDERSTANDING THE DIFFERENT TYPES OF DENTIST

Every dentist who qualifies leaves Dental School with a degree in dentistry, and then they must register with the General Dental Council. Some dentists do general dentistry all their career. Others dentists go on to do advanced qualifications to become more competent in different areas of dentistry. Some do specialist training and exams, and then go onto the specialist register of the General Dental Council. Some dentists become mainly academics.

There are many fields of dentistry, however there is no category for a *Specialist in Dental Implants*.

General dentists and specialist dentists, such as Oral Surgeons, Prosthodontists, Periodontists, Restorative Specialists, can all train to place implants.

Now listen closely.

Some General Dentists and Specialists are both highly trained and experienced in dental implants. Conversely, some General Dentists and Specialists have had little training or experience.

I know, now I'm confusing you! Stay with me, because all will become clear.

Some *general* dentists may have more training and experience in dental implant placement and restoring, than some *specialists* may and visa-versa.

All in all, this makes it difficult to know who to trust with your surgery. So, let's look at some of the questions you can be asking.

THE TOP 10 QUESTIONS TO ASK AN IMPLANT SURGEON

Which qualifications in implant dentistry do you have?

The *Diploma* in Implant Dentistry from the Royal College of Surgeons is considered to be a gold standard qualification in Implant Dentistry in the U.K. The diploma covers placing simple implants.
The *Advanced* Diploma in Implant Dentistry from the Royal College of Surgeons covers more advanced techniques of bone grafting, advanced implant placement and restoring dental implants.

How many implants have you placed in total, and how many in the last 12 months?

A starting point in skill is experience. How many implants has the surgeon placed in total? To give you an idea of numbers, our surgeon, Dr Adam Glassford, is one of the leading implant surgeons in the country, and he has placed over 5000 implants.

Some highly regarded Implantologists are suggesting that an implant surgeon should be placing a minimum of 50 implants per year to maintain their skills. If a surgeon hasn't placed many recently, then their skills could be rusty. To give you an idea of numbers, Adam Glassford is placing about 500 implants each year.

Every surgeon has to start somewhere, of course. The way a new surgeon starts is with a competent and experienced mentor. This mentor will be a skilled senior surgeon who will be by their side for their first procedures, perhaps up to the first 50 procedures.

Will you do the surgery and also restore?

To 'restore' means to fit the top part of the implant onto the fixture, the restoration which is the implant crown/bridge/denture.

There are two main stages when having an implant placed: the surgical fixture placement and then the fitting of the top part, the restoration.

These stages can both be done by the same clinician or can be done by two clinicians - a surgeon and a restorative dentist working together.

Sometimes advanced bone grafting is required, and this could be provided by a more experienced surgeon first, then the implant fixture placed by the less experienced surgeon. Any of these options is fine, however each clinician needs to be competent in each aspect and the team needs to be experienced in working together.

Historically, some surgeons with little restorative experience placed implant fixtures. Without skilled restorative knowledge, some of these fixtures were placed into optimum bone, however were placed in such a difficult position for the restorative dentist to restore, that the aesthetics of the final result would be very poor. So, the implant fixtures needed removing and replacing to fix the aesthetic issues. Not good.

There have also been instances of great surgery by one clinician, however followed by poor placement of the restoration by an inexperienced restorative clinician. Poor restorative placement can result in overloading of biting forces, which can cause failure.

In these cases, where there are several clinicians involved, in the case of failure, *who is ultimately responsible*? This is a question that you need to ask of each of those clinicians before treatment starts. It gets more complicated when there are more clinicians involved.

Simple is good.

There is a balance between optimum position of the implant fixtures in relation to being in the best bone and optimum position of the aesthetics of the final restoration. In my personal opinion, the ideal is to find one clinician who is highly experienced in everything: bone grafting, implant surgery and highly experienced in cosmetic dentistry.

Which implant system do you use?

Take this as an analogy. Choosing an implant manufacturer is a little like choosing a brand of a car.

There are different car manufacturers. Some are cheaper, some more expensive. Some manufacturers are renowned for reliability, enhanced safety features and research into technology. Some not.

Some manufacturers give a 3-year warranty. Some 10 years.

Some manufacturers go out of business and leave you with no access to spare parts. Some manufacturers are based only in one country, and if you needed a part in another country, then you would struggle to access a mechanic who knew the brand of car or who could locate spare parts.

In a similar way, there are many implant systems, but not all are equal. In the last decade, dental implants have become a standard treatment in dentistry, and there are many types being offered by various dental implant companies. But are they offering the same quality, and have these systems been clinically proven in long-term studies? There are critical differences between implant systems. There are cheap imported systems on the market that may not have even been tested in humans!

Are you getting the picture?

A good implant system will

- comply with internationally accepted quality standards
- have long-term documented clinical research
- be available in many countries, so that if you were to move abroad, then you could easily find a clinician that uses the same system
- have a long-term manufacturer's guarantee
- give a commitment from the manufacturer that they will continue to make components to older implants over the coming years, so that 'parts' will be available in case of the rare event that a component needs replacing.

We use a world leader in implant manufacturing, Straumann, and this is why. Only few systems on the market have been scientifically tested. The Straumann Dental Implant System is one of the best documented, with more than 35 years of extensive scientific, clinical evidence and support by more than 700 scientific publications.

As a pioneer and global leader in implant dentistry, Straumann have been researching, developing and manufacturing implants since 1974. In collaboration with renowned international clinics, research institutes and universities, they have pioneered many ground-breaking technologies in implant dentistry.

More than 14 million Straumann implants have been placed worldwide in over 70 countries. We like the Swiss precision engineering and commitment to clinical excellence.

Do you take a CBCT scan?

The gold standard in Implant Dentistry today is to use 3D CBCT for every implant placement.

Regular 2D x-rays just cannot show 3 dimensionally how much bone there is, and can give false positives, showing bone height but not width. CBCT scanning clearly shows the surgeon how much bone there is, where the arteries and veins are positioned, and crucially, where the nerves lie. The surgeon can place to the nearest millimetre, increasing safety of the procedure to almost 100%.

I must stress to you that it is essential that your surgeon takes a CT scan.

No scan? Walk away.

What is your success rate?

Dental implants are one of the most successful surgical procedures. The average success rate is about 96-98%.

Every implant surgeon should have statistics on their success rate. Ideally, you want a surgeon who has placed thousands of implants with a very high success rate.

As an example, our surgeon, Dr Adam Glassford, has a 98.8% success rate and has placed over 5000 implants.

What's the guarantee?

Now you might presume that surgical procedures do not carry a guarantee.

Well interestingly, dental implants have such a high success rate, that surgeons are able to give a guarantee. A confident surgeon will give a clear guarantee on their work.

Remember there are two parts to the dental implant - and two parts to a guarantee.

1. The implant fixture guarantee

We work with our dental implant manufacturer for many reasons, and one good reason is that they give a *lifetime* guarantee on the implant fixtures that we use. If a Straumann implant fixture was to fail, then Straumann will supply any Straumann surgeon worldwide (not just your initial surgeon), with a replacement fixture for you free of charge. For full Ts and Cs, see **www.straumann.co.uk**.

We have heard of inferior quality implant systems where the implant fixture actually fractured under the stress of loading when biting. You guessed.....this manufacturer didn't provide a guarantee.

We have also seen other manufacturers discontinue lines of implants, so if the restoration was to need replacing in the future, then the clinician is unable to acquire the part, so the whole implant had to be removed and replaced.

We have also had people come to ask for our help with failing implants provided abroad. However, there is no record of the implant system used as it was so obscure or had gone out of business, and again, the implants had to be removed and the whole procedure started again.

As well as keeping the information logged at our clinic, we give our patients an 'Implant Passport' at the end of treatment. This shows precisely which implant components were used. So, if in the event that a different surgeon needed to continue the aftercare anywhere in the world, then the information is there.

2. The guarantee by the surgeon

This is a different guarantee which covers the surgery, crown, bridge or denture and is made by the surgeon and practice delivering your implant care. A confident surgeon may give up to 5-years' guarantee; however, this is normally subject to a patient's commitment to maintaining good oral hygiene and having regular follow-up visits.

Remember, amazing dental implant treatment can still fail if a patient does not clean around the implant properly. So, check the terms and conditions of every guarantee thoroughly, to fully understand your own responsibility.

Do you offer sedation?

Some clinicians don't offer sedation, and that shouldn't be a problem for a confident patient having simple surgery. However, more nervous patients and some complex procedures can be much more comfortable with sedation.

Ok, let me rephrase that and let's be honest. Some big bone grafting and multiple implant cases are significant surgical procedures for a patient. With sedation, they become easy. Do you remember that sedation has an amnesic effect?

Personally, I think having the option of sedation is important.

Sometimes the surgeon may provide the sedation themselves, and sometimes a second clinician is there to provide it. Either is fine.

What after care do you provide?

A great implant team will have a great after-care package. We know that success is mainly down to the care of the implants after treatment.

Are hygiene appointments recommended – or better still, compulsory?

Are annual reviews highly recommended?

If an implant surgeon just wants to do the procedure as quickly as possible and never wants to see you again, well I think that we can all hear the warning sirens and see the red flashing lights.

Can I see examples of your work?

It is vital that you ask to see examples of the work produced by an implant dentist. They should be delighted to show off their amazing work, and be more than happy to show you many, many cases of photos and x-rays illustrating the before and after results of their work.

You want to be able to say, wow, they look like gorgeous real teeth.

Different clinicians have different restorative styles too. Some love bright Hollywood white teeth, whereas some prefer the natural look, and others appear to have little interest in what their patients' teeth look like! A great clinician will be able to give every patient what they are looking for. They will show you different styles and colours of beautiful teeth, which reflect the different preferences of their patients.

If a clinician doesn't have any cases to show you, or you have any doubts over the aesthetics, just walk away and find one who does.

TOP TIP

When looking at before and after cases, take a really careful look at the gum margins on the after photos. Are they pink and healthy, or are they red, swollen and sore? Gums should look pink, healthy and firm. This is a very big clue as to how good the work is.

Reviews

Recommendations and reviews form an important part of life now and are interesting when taken as part of the overall picture.

However, we all know that some companies have average products and are amazing at acquiring reviews. Whereas some, perhaps niche companies, spend more effort on their amazing products than asking for reviews. So, take a balanced view.

A Note About Membership of Organisations

Dentists may be members of many organisations and whilst such organisations often provide excellent courses for dentists to attend, any dentist can pay for membership and join them. So, remember that this is not a qualification. Let's not take memberships as a sign of experience or quality. Although it can be a good sign of the clinician's keenness to keep up to date, and it may be a worry if they are not a member of any organisations at all.

The Association of Dental Implantology (ADI) is a study group where Implantologists meet to further their knowledge of dental implant care. The ADI produces guidelines on best practice in the field of implantology are ideal to be used in day to day practice and our Implant Team are members and love the up-to-date information and teaching that they receive.

Finally

And only now, after getting all the really important information, ask about price.

Only now can you compare real value.

SUMMARY OF THE TOP 10 QUESTIONS TO ASK AN IMPLANT SURGEON

1. Which qualifications in implant dentistry do you have?

2. How many implants have you placed in total, and how many implants have you placed in the last 12 months?

3. Will you do the surgery and also restore?

4. Which implant system do you use?

5. Do you take a CBCT scan?

6. What is your success rate?

7. What's the guarantee? And what are the terms and conditions?

8. Do you offer sedation?

9. What after care do you provide?

10. Can I see examples of your work?

"I am so, so glad I had it done. It's changed my whole life."

SHIRLEY HARTON

PATIENT OF DR ADAM GLASSFORD

PLANNING YOUR
WHOLE SMILE

Have you seen a smile where no two teeth seem to match? There are crowns and fillings of different shapes and colours, and the gums are different heights. The result is just untidy.

I call this *patch-work dentistry*. One item of dentistry is done every few years and the result is a patchwork appearance. If you have a new implant placed, are you just adding to the patchwork? It is time to take a step back and look at your whole smile, so the size, shape and colour of your new implant can be planned with your whole smile in mind.

Before you start treatment, let us consider your smile as a whole. Is there any other work that needs to be considered together with your implant treatment?

Let's look holistically at your smile right now. Grab a mirror and let's take a look closely.

The smile is made up of:

1. gums
2. teeth
3. lips

Your Gums

- Are your gums pink and healthy?
- Is your gum line symmetrical?
- Do you have a gummy smile?

Your Teeth

- Are you happy with the shade of white of your teeth, or would you like them whiter?
- Are all your teeth a good shape, symmetrical and even?
- Are your teeth crowded or spaced? Would you like them correcting with straightening?
- Do you have old crowns and fillings that need changing for aesthetic restorations?
- Are any of your teeth worn or chipped?

Your Lips

- Are you happy with the shape of your lips, or are they thin or asymmetrical due to teeth that are irregular or set back in the smile, and therefore not supporting your lips well?

All these aspects need discussing at the planning stage, so that your case can be planned to get your desired result.

There may need to be a *multi-disciplinary* team approach.

Multi-disciplinary means that different clinicians with different skills plan your care together. They work side by side to give you the best outcome. A highly skilled implant surgeon may not be the best clinician to also provide highly technical aesthetic dentistry or treat crowded teeth, for example. The best result, in this example, may be for an implant surgeon, aesthetic dentist and orthodontist to plan your care and work together holistically.

There are different looks for different people. Let's look at some examples.

THE NATURAL LOOK

Some patients want to keep the look of their existing smile. So missing teeth are replaced to match in with the remaining teeth, matching the colour and reflecting the nuances of aging teeth.

Take a look at the smile below. This patient has a missing front tooth. The other incisor has recession at the root, showing as darker yellow. In this photo, the implant fixture has been placed, which we can see just showing in the gum. The gum has healed, and the implant is ready to be restored with an implant-crown.

Let's look at the aesthetics of the other natural front tooth. There is recession at the gum line, with the yellower dentine showing, and the tip of this incisor is very slightly worn. The teeth have a natural yellow hue.

The patient requested the new implant crown match her existing teeth and this was what was provided.

REAL EXAMPLE: CASE 1

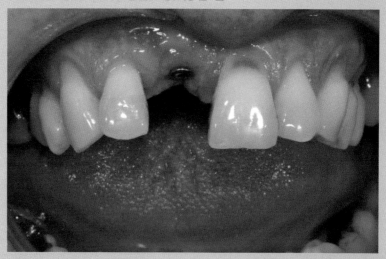

Case 1: before. The implant crown was created by the ceramists to mimic the matching incisor as perfectly as possible. The implant crown has the appearance of recession, being shaded darker at the gum line, and the biting edge of the tooth is created to look slightly worn.

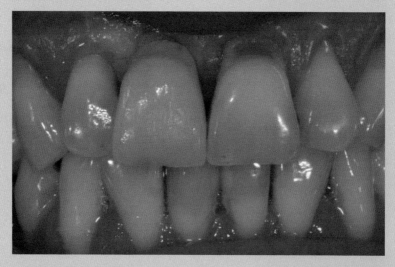

Case 1: after treatment. The implant crown has been fitted to the implant fixture. Case by Dr Adam Glassford.

REAL EXAMPLE: CASE 2

In this second example, which of the two incisors is the implant crown?

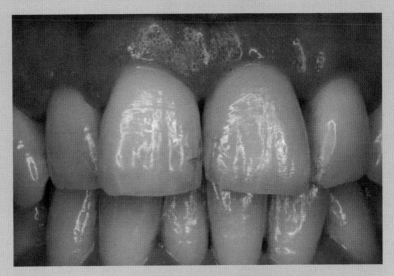

It is difficult to tell. Actually, it is the front right incisor, as you are looking at the photo. Case by Dr Adam Glassford.

Let's look at a more complex case.

REAL EXAMPLE: CASE 3

THE SMILE MAKEOVER

Take a close look at this next smile.

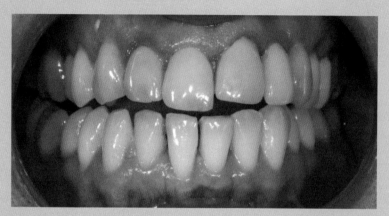

You can't see it in the photo, but this lady had a failing front tooth that needed replacement with a dental implant. She could just have had this tooth replaced and matched to the teeth either side. However, she didn't like the teeth either side. She wanted to review the overall aesthetics of her smile. So, this was discussed at the planning stage.

Let's look at her aesthetic issues of the upper teeth.

Concerns:

- o Gums: asymmetry of the upper gumline
- o Colour of the teeth: natural yellow. A whiter colour was preferred, yet still within the natural-looking range
- o Shape of the teeth: asymmetrical teeth, including all the upper 8 front teeth showing most in the smile
- o Centre-line: not straight
- o The edges/tips of the front 6 upper front teeth were out of line, especially the front incisors

There were four old crowns on the upper front teeth, with one of those failing and needing replacing with a dental implant crown.

So, the plan in order:

1. Removal of the failing tooth and a temporary restoration placed.
2. Professional Teeth Whitening treatment of the remaining natural teeth during the healing period.
3. Placement of the dental implant fixture, with adjustment of the gum-line to create symmetry.
4. After the healing period, placement of new crowns/implant-crown/veneers on the upper 8 front teeth - all at the same time.

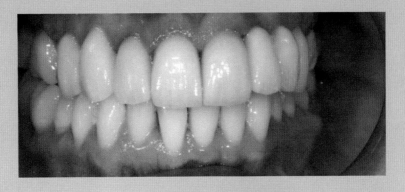

Case 3: after
Treatment by Dr Adam Glassford

Note: At every stage the patient had temporary restorations so she could smile with confidence.

HARMONY OF COLOUR

When ceramists make crowns and veneers, then they build up each layer of the porcelain in a similar way to the colours of a natural tooth. They start with a darker layer, mimicking dentine, then a middle lighter layer, mimicking enamel and place a translucent layer too. It really is art. Many, many colours are used in the layering process.

To recreate a matching crown to one already in place, is like asking an artist to recreate an oil painting exactly to match one painted previously. Possible, but almost impossible. It is much more accurate to create works of art at the same time, side by side. In the same way, the results of ceramists are much more consistent if adjacent crowns/veneers are created at the same time.

Creating all of these 8 crowns/veneers in the photo above at the same time ensured that all would match. They were colour-matched to the newly whitened lower teeth.

Let's look at another complex case.

REAL EXAMPLE: CASE 4

This patient had old crowns which had recession at the roots, shown by the dark lines near the gum. Also, the tips of the teeth were uneven and presented in a 'Negative Smile-line.' She needed one failing tooth replacing with a dental implant.

The patient asked to redress all of the issues in the smile at the same time.

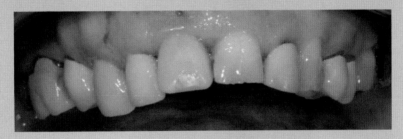

Before

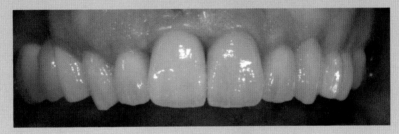

After

Full smile redesign, including new implant and additional crowns.

Case by Dr Adam Glassford.

REAL EXAMPLE: CASE 5

DENTAL IMPLANTS REPLACING A FAILING DENTAL BRIDGE

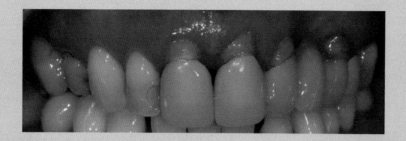

Before: Note the failing dental bridge with severe recession around it, and the bone loss around the canine on the right side of the photo.

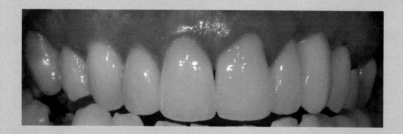

After: The dental bridge was replaced with a dental implant bridge and the old crowns replaced at the same time, so that the restorations match.

Case by Dr Adam Glassford.

REAL EXAMPLE: CASE 6

REPLACING FAILING UPPER TEETH AND OLD PARTIAL DENTURE WITH IMPLANT-RETAINED LOCATORS

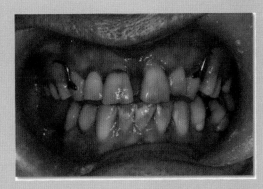

Before: The six upper front teeth were failing, with gum disease, and the patient was wearing a partial denture, replacing all the back teeth.

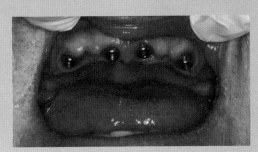

During treatment: The remaining upper teeth were removed, and four dental implant fixtures placed.

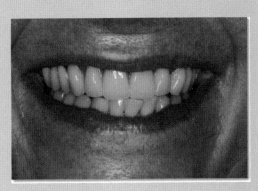

After: The lower teeth were whitened with professional teeth whitening, and the upper teeth were restored with an implant-retained denture fixed to the implants.

A Note About Professional Teeth Whitening

Teeth Whitening only works on enamel, not on dental-made restorations. It is so important to choose the colour of your teeth before any treatment is started. If a natural yellow crown made is made to match your naturally yellow teeth, then if you were to whiten your natural teeth, the crown would remain the same colour. Yellow.

So, whiten your teeth first then have any new crowns made to match the whiter colour. You will avoid expensive remakes.

Stacey's Story

"When I was a dental nurse, a lady in her late 60s came to visit us complaining of ill-fitting dentures. She was unable to wear them. In fact, she actually arrived to the appointment with no teeth in at all, not wearing any dentures. She proceeded to pull 6 pairs of previously-made dentures out a plastic bag with that she couldn't wear.

She was quite depressed and not confident at all. She came across as quite moody, almost to the point of being aggressive. It turned out her husband had passed away a few years ago and since then she had not socialised with any of her family or friends. The fact that she could not wear her dentures even to talk, let alone eat, mortified her. Her health was deteriorating due to living on a soft diet as she was unable to chew her food properly. All this led to her suffering with mild depression.

We discussed an over-denture on implants and she loved the idea. We proceeded with the surgery and successfully fitted upper and lower implant-retained dentures.

We called her back after 6 months for a review.

This is why the memory stays with me…. the same lady literally skipped into the practice. Her hair was freshly permed, her face was made-up beautifully with bright red lipstick and a smile as wide as you would ever imagine.
She began to thank us for changing her life. She went on to explain that she now is constantly out visiting

friends and family. She can now confidently talk without having to worry about a lisp or her teeth falling out!

What was also amazing, was that her health had dramatically improved as her diet was no longer mainly soft foods. She had been able to introduce roughage into her daily diet. Her mental health had improved and she was no longer taking medication for depression. Her overall quality of life had changed dramatically.

Seeing this first hand, made me love my job and dental implants more and more.

I now work for one of the world leaders in implant manufacturing and I am able to share my experiences and passion of why dental implants are simply life-changing."

STACEY SAGAR,

STRAUMANN

YORKSHIRE AND HUMBERSIDE TERRITORY MANAGER

Shirley's Story

"When I was younger, I'd always had really nice teeth, but over the years, they got worse and worse, until my teeth looked so bad and felt so wobbly, they felt like they were all going to fall out. I was always so conscious of what I could eat when I went out for meals. I was paranoid that I would knock one of them out. I couldn't bite at the front and they were flaring out. The last year before I had my teeth sorted, in photos, you would not see my teeth. I didn't smile.

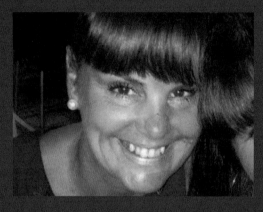

It was overtaking my life and I hated them.

It got to the stage when I was so down about it.
I never thought I'd be able to afford implants. You read all these different things and I thought there's no way I can afford that. I thought I'd need one implant per tooth and knew how expensive that might be, but I didn't realise that there are many different options.

Anyway, my dentist referred me. Before I came in, I said to my husband, I bet I can't have implants as I didn't want to get my hopes up.
When I came to the implant consultation, I felt quite anxious and worked up. Then everything was explained. I asked: "So I can have implants?" and Dr Glassford said yes! I just couldn't believe it and I was on a high. Then it was discussed that I could have

them on finance, I couldn't believe that I could afford them either. At the end of this same year, they will be paid for.

First, I had to have all of my old (failing) teeth out. I had all my treatment under sedation, and that was great. I just remember Adam talking to me, then remember just as he was finishing. But It didn't register having to have so many teeth out, that your gums swell. I was in bed for a full day. It took about 5 days for the swelling to go down, then the immediate denture fit, and I loved it.

I remember a week after that first appointment, I never looked back.

If anyone was in a similar situation to me, I would tell them not to panic, just give yourself a few days after your old teeth have been taken out. Just give your mouth time to let the swelling go down. Taking teeth out is worse than putting them back in! Having my old teeth out was the worst part of the whole procedure. After this all the treatment was brilliant.

When I had the implants placed, I don't remember anything about that because of sedation!

Now I have my implants, I feel a million times better. It's given me a whole new lease of life. I love having my photo taking. I can go into a restaurant and have anything I want to eat

It has made a difference to my confidence. Before, I used to feel that people were looking at my bad teeth.

Now people say, "Your teeth are mint, we can't stop looking at them!" My family are so proud of me.

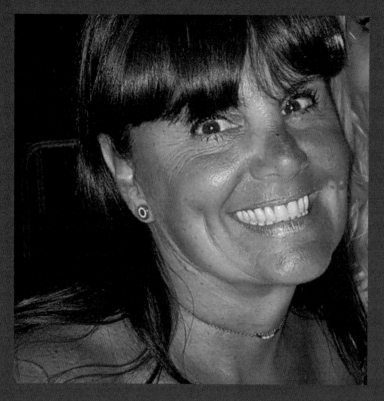

There is no soreness now. There is nothing that I can't eat.

I am so, so glad I had it done.
It's changed my whole life."

SHIRLEY HARTON

PATIENT OF DR ADAM GLASSFORD

"Always ask for answers, and keep asking until you understand. "

FOUR BIG QUESTIONS

QUESTION ONE: ARE IMPLANTS CHEAPER ABROAD?

have to admit, it's really tempting, isn't it? Travel to a sun-kissed, far-flung place and have cheap treatment, a hotel recovery, fly home and all done.

But is it that simple?

Online adverts point out the cost savings but in the long term, is this really going to save you money?

As a national referral centre for dental implants in the UK, we often see the consequences of *dental tourism.* Patients have been abroad to have cheap dental work carried out, return with problems and ask us for help to sort them out.

As clinicians we feel very strongly about this. So please listen to us carefully.

We see lovely patients, who have taken their hard-earned money to try and find good value abroad. And we are seeing dental implant placement and restorations that are of a significantly lower quality than we would expect to see placed by experienced surgeons in the UK. Sometimes the placement is so poor that the patient cannot even clean around the implants. And we see restorations of such poor aesthetic finish that the whole treatment, including all the implant fixtures, needs removing and starting from the beginning.

Devastating.

Dentists and laboratories in the UK comply with strict cross infection and quality controls which don't apply to some parts of the world.

Any dentist can place implants after just a weekend "implant course." How do patients know how experienced a foreign surgeon is?

When we plan implants with a patient, often they need hygiene coaching for several weeks or months to achieve great oral hygiene ready for implant placement to be 100% successful. We are hearing of patients turning up at foreign clinics and being given implant surgery regardless of the condition of the oral hygiene. No wonder these implants are failing!

Implant fixtures normally need time to 'osseointegrate' before the final restoration is placed on top. Sometimes a temporary restoration can be placed immediately, however, a permanent restoration is normally placed later. Osseointegration takes 2-3 months. Grafted bone takes 3+ months to heal before loading. Immediate loading is not suitable in every case, and if loaded too soon, then failure occurs.

We have seen so many implant tourism disaster stories, that we could cry with the patients who come asking for help.

Patients who truly believed they are getting good value, find themselves in a situation of failure with no follow up or recourse. It would take multiple foreign trips abroad for their original surgeon to replace the work. However, some foreign surgeons are not giving guarantees and are accepting no responsibility. Their patients have nowhere to appeal for justice. They are left out of pocket, in pain and needing all the work replacing.

Good implant dentistry normally takes many appointments over several weeks and months.

A quick fix can be the quick route to failure.

What about aftercare and supervision? That takes a life time. A life time of trips abroad? Is that feasible? The cost of returning to a foreign country for follow-up over a life-time is massive.

There are over 130 different dental implant systems worldwide and each has their own unique set of tools and components. Many of the cheaper dental implant systems do not comply with the strict rules of the UK and so are not available here. We have seen failing work carried out abroad that cannot be repaired here because the system that has been used is no longer supported or cannot be sourced in the UK. This leaves the patient unable to have ongoing maintenance for their implant work in the event of problems, leaving them with the choice of returning to the country that the work was originally provided, or having the failing work removed and the procedure started over again.

Still tempted to have a dental procedure done abroad?

Perhaps take a moment to think again. It can work out much more expensive in the long-run.

QUESTION TWO: ARE YOU SUITABLE FOR DENTAL IMPLANTS?

Let's talk about you.

There are six questions to ask here.

Question 1: Do you have enough bone?

Bone levels are assessed with the 3D CT scanner, where the height and width of the bone can be accurately measured.

Historically, implants were long and wide, and needed a lot of bone. The thinking was that the longer and wider, then the stronger the implant would be. However, with more research, new technology and more advanced materials, smaller, new-generation implants have been found to work just as well, if not actually better.

Some of the more cutting-edge implants available now only need 5mm of bone depth. They are tiny and incredibly strong.

So even if you have lost a lot of bone already, then you may still have enough bone already to have implants placed. But what about those people who don't have enough bone already?

If so much bone volume has been lost, that even one of these small implants are too large, then there are modern techniques of bone grafting available, as discussed earlier.

Remember: it is simpler and cheaper to have dental implants immediately after tooth extraction when there is maximum bone, however if you have already lost a lot of bone, then there are amazing techniques available.

However, there are a few – very few – cases, where it is impossible to reconstruct the jaw as there has been devastating bone loss in the jaw. There simply is not enough bone to provide grafting, or not enough volume of gum over the bone to leave room to place grafting and close the surgical site. Approximately 1% of patients in our experience fall into this group.

This is why there is a clock ticking after tooth extraction. Time is important.

So, don't accept a quick diagnosis of "there's not enough bone for dental implants" until you have had a consultation with a leading dental implant surgeon who is highly experienced in complex grafting procedures. To them, your case could be simple. Chances are you are one of the 99% of patients who are suitable for dental implants.

Question 2: Are you well enough?

For success, dental implants need to be accepted by the body, so that *osseointegration* can take place. There are a few medical conditions that affect our immune system and affect our ability of our body to 'accept' a foreign body and therefore affect implant surgery.

Some of these conditions only temporarily affect the immune system, so implants can be placed after these existing circumstances have changed, for example:

- Smoking, alcoholism and drug addiction. Wait until dependency has stopped.

- Pregnancy. Wait until after childbirth

- Growing children. Wait until after the growing stage is complete, so normally after the age of 18-21.

- Uncontrolled diabetes increases the risk of infection and has a longer healing time. Wait until the diabetes is controlled well.

- Illness requiring anticoagulants (blood thinners). Liaison with the medical doctor is necessary to see if they can be stopped or changed before and during surgery.

- Autoimmune diseases (e.g.: lupus, rheumatoid arthritis, etc.) lead to a longer healing time. Wait until in remission.

- Untreated psychiatric or psychological problems. This can compromise the security of the team or the patient during the procedure, the patient may have dissatisfaction with the final result because of unrealistic expectations and be unable to care for the final implants.

- Other diseases, for example, severe sinusitis, septacaemia. Wait until resolved.

- Some conditions permanently subdue the immune system, so implants will never be suitable, these include:

    - osteoporosis and other bone diseases

    - cardiovascular disease (e.g. recent myocardial infarction, valvular disease, heart failure)

    - long-term treatment with anti-rejection drugs that suppress or slow down the immune system

- o cancer that is not in remission, has been treated with bisphosphonates or required radiotherapy treatments in the jaw area

- o HIV or AIDS

Question 3: Are you too old?

Simply, no.

Guess how old the oldest implant patient is that we know of in the UK?

> "We just put an implant in a 101-year-old, last week. He found it absolutely fine. Wished he'd done it years ago."
> Kate Keating, Straumann.

Question 4: Is your mouth healthy enough?

Any existing infections in the mouth need to be treated. Gum disease needs treating and any tooth infections near the site of the implant need treating before surgery. If they were not treated, then these infections would affect the implant and its success.

Question 5: Do you smoke?

Smoking reduces your ability to heal, so you need to stop smoking. Forever. If not, then your implant will probably fail.

Smoking has a dramatic effect on the health of your mouth as well as any dental implant work that may be planned. Apart from the overall risks of cancer within the mouth, throat and lungs, healing from any surgery is reduced. Smoking means that your blood is able to carry less oxygen and this means that healing tissues don't repair as quickly or as well. The effect on dental implants in the extreme can be total failure of the implants to bond to the bone.

Even in light smokers, 5-15 per day, the success rate of implants reduces from around 98% to around 90%.

In heavy smokers, 15+ per day, the success rate reduces to below 80%.

In patients smoking over 30 cigarettes per day, implants are totally contra-indicated as the failure rate is unacceptably high.

Smoking also contributes to bone loss around both natural teeth and implants.

Smoking is strongly associated with a condition called 'peri-implantitis' where bone is lost around dental implants.

My advice to any smoker is to give up completely. After 3 months of not smoking, the blood oxygen levels will be back to that of a non-smoker and healing will be normal. If smoking is avoided long-term, the success rate of implants will continue to be as high as someone who has never smoked. You may wish to discuss smoking cessation clinics with your local doctor.

Question 6: Are you motivated for the after care?

Implants need caring for just like natural teeth. Every day, the gum around the implant fixture needs cleaning with interdental brushes and floss.

Every single day.

Twice a day.

No exceptions or your gorgeous new implants will probably fail.

This may be a serious turnaround for you. The reason your natural teeth may have failed, could have been from lack of dental care of your natural teeth. If you don't care for implants, then they too may fail.

Let's hear what Chris has to say. I think you find it interesting. Really interesting.

Chris's Story

"All my life, I've never had good teeth. I have never been confident to smile. My teeth were in an embarrassing state due to smoking. By the time I'd realised I'd got a problem with my teeth, it was a big problem – gum disease! I'd attended a dentist every six months, but I was never told that I had any problems with my gums.

Then I needed referring to the dental hospital in Sheffield for one particular tooth. I was told it wasn't a problem with just that one tooth, it was all my teeth! I had gaps developing between some of my teeth which I was self-conscious about, and my gums were red and inflamed.

I decided that something needed to be done about it and I spent a year researching.

I liked the approach of "get rid of the problem, let it all heal and then restore" rather than rushing the treatment. I had been as far as Scotland and London for appointments, but I didn't feel comfortable. I even researched different implant systems.

I felt comfortable with the fact that you wanted to do the work *properly* rather than *quickly*, and I liked that you work so efficiently.

I am now very caring about my smile and oral hygiene. Yes, it's not cheap, but the results speak for themselves. It changes your psychology– not putting your hand over your mouth.

Implants have made me more outgoing and confident as a person. I am not embarrassed to smile now and I have become a more positive person.

Once you've had the work for a couple of weeks, they feel like they are natural teeth – part of yourself.

I was so ashamed of what my teeth used to be like. I know that implants gave me a second chance of having a good smile. They have properly changed my life."

CHRIS BROOKES

PATIENT OF DR ADAM GLASSFORD

QUESTION THREE: HOW SAFE ARE DENTAL IMPLANTS?

When provided by an experienced surgeon, dental implants are one of the safest surgical procedures with one of the highest success rates.

However as with any surgery, in the wrong hands, the risks are high. Remember 'cheap' rarely means 'quality.'

A highly trained and experienced clinician will make a correct diagnosis from the beginning, plans the treatment with precision and is skilled in executing the treatment.

An ethical clinician puts you as the patient first before anything else.

It is estimated that 98% of implant treatments are successful. Success means no long-lasting complications and the implant remains healthy and functional.

So, let's take a look at those 2% of cases that fail. What can go wrong and why?

The implant fixture may not *osseointegrate*, meaning that the bone does not bond to the fixture.

This is rare. However, it does happen. There is rarely any pain, just that the implant becomes loose and eventually falls out. To re-treat this case, then the failed implant would need removing, if still in position, then the site left to heal. The causes for failure would need to be identified and addressed, then another implant would normally be placed.

So, let's look at the three main causes for failure.

1. Planning Failure

Your surgeon will assess the quality of the bone, looking at how dense it is, and the volume. This is done through 3D CT scanning. Then the surgeon will plan how the implant will be placed, whether additional bone is needed, and how soon the implant can be loaded, meaning how fast can you start really biting on it.

If the surgeon overloads an implant too soon before healing is complete, or places too few implants in a situation when they will get overloaded, then the implants may fail.

With good mentoring of training-surgeons and digital scanning technology, this should be rare.

2. Patient Failure

You, the patient, have to understand what your responsibility is.

You must do what your surgeon asks, clean around the implant religiously, have implant checks every year, visit your hygienist as regularly as recommended.

You must not lie! Don't lie about your medical condition or say you don't smoke if you do. There's no point. Your implants could fail simply because of you.

3. Surgical Failure

The 3D CBCT scan (CT xray) shows where the nerves and blood vessels are, so that the surgeon can plan where to place the implant. The surgeon can guide the implant into place in exactly the right position to the nearest millimetre.

Before 3D CBCT scanning, there was an increased risk that the surgeon could place an implant in the wrong place, into a nerve for example, and numbness of the tongue and lip could occur, which could be permanent. With a 3D CBCT scan and good planning, this should never happen nowadays.

Remember the rule, if the surgeon doesn't do a CBCT scan at the planning stage, then walk away. There is no excuse for poor surgical planning.

Implants are one of the safest surgical procedures that you can have, yet why is there still a nation of people who are struggling with loose dentures and missing teeth?

QUESTION FOUR: WHY ARE MORE PEOPLE NOT HAVING DENTAL IMPLANTS?

Now this is a very interesting question. We have spent a lot of time trying to understand this.

We see such life-changing results at our clinic, that we find it incomprehensible that more people are not having dental implants.

If more people knew all the information surrounding missing teeth, with the subsequent bone loss, the problems of dentures and dental-bridges, and more importantly the loss of biting ability leading to reduced nutrition and the reduction in self-confidence, then I think that more people would choose to have dental implants.

So, let's look at these issues more closely.

A Mystery

Until quite recently, dental implants have been a big mystery both to patients and older-generation dentists.

For hundreds of years, dentures were the acceptable solution for replacement for missing teeth. Dentists are still taught in dental school that dentures are the mainstream method of replacing missing teeth. However, also taught at dental school are the compounding issues that dentures have on the remaining teeth and dental health. Yet dentures are still being churned out in their millions each year. Why is this?

Interestingly, the UK population is lagging behind many developed countries in dental implant treatment. Presently, only approx. 0.3% of the UK adults have implants, whereas other countries have much higher density. Over 6% of the adults in South Korea and Israel, have implants, and almost 3% of adults in Spain and Italy have implants.

One reason that the statistics in the UK are so low could be our *NHS mind-set*.

However necessary dental implants are, the NHS is simply unable to afford the cost of dental implants for the whole of the UK population with so many missing teeth. A rough estimate is that there are 300 million missing teeth in adults in England and Wales alone, as statistics show that on average, each adult has 6 missing teeth. The NHS is simply unable to afford offering dental implants as a mainstream treatment. (Note that the NHS offers implants in extreme cases, such as post-jaw resection following cancer treatment.)

However, times have changed. Our mind-set is changing.

People are living longer and longer.

The modern savvy consumer easily expects to live into their 80s and 90s with good health and nutrition. We are demanding an increased standard in the quality of living.

We are not content with old-fashioned, antiquated solutions such as dentures. We are more aware of modern procedures, and now implant treatment is now on the rise. Even in the UK.

The Issue of Fear

Many people are fearful of the dentist. They had difficult experiences. If a patient has many missing teeth, then that means that they have endured many extractions. This memory can be overwhelming and difficult to move beyond.

However modern dentistry is different. There are dental teams who are lovely, welcoming and adore their patients.

There are ways to make every treatment gentle. There is the magically relaxing sedation.

I've said this before, and I will say it one more time. Keep looking until you find a dental team that you enjoy being with and who you trust. Find a team that offers sedation. We think it makes all the difference.

Lack of Knowledge

We consider this to be another key reason that more people don't have dental implants. Simply people don't understand fully about them. They don't know about the long-term benefits. They don't understand how devastating missing teeth, dentures and dental bridges can be. They don't understand that initially dental implants are the most expensive, yet in the long-term, they are the best value by miles. This is exactly why we have written this book.

Now you know.

"Since a cycle accident when I was aged 7, I have had many crowns for my front two teeth. Over the years, as the need to replace took its toll on my bone and gum line, my confidence in smiling, laughing and eating declined. I got used to hiding behind my hand, half-smiling and missed apples!

Five implants later, the change is amazing. I look like I would have done without that accident over 40 years ago! You have changed my life."

NICK

PATIENT OF DR ADAM GLASSFORD.

"The real question is this. What is the cost of not having implants?"

THE WORRY OF COST

Yes, I do think that one of the biggest issues is the cost of dental implants. The immediate cost. However, I have one question first for you to keep in your mind.

What is the cost of *not* having implants?

We are now going to look at the immediate and long-term price comparisons of options after losing a tooth. Follow me really carefully. I want you to fully understand the implications of tooth loss. I'm going to ask you to be patient with me as I approximate costs to make this really important point.

Imagine a woman called Holly loses one of her premolars due to decay. A common scenario.

Let's say that Holly is 40 and works in a marketing company. Now Holly has four options to replace her missing tooth. Let's look at these more closely.

HOLLY'S OPTION 1

Do nothing and leave the gap.

Initial cost £0.

However, leaving a gap has embarrassing social implications and if the teeth next to the gap start to drift into the space, then more gaps can open up, compounding the problem. Holly may become less confident socially and professionally and this may impact her job. According to the research that we have looked at, Holly has a high risk of becoming a little more reclusive. She may cover her mouth when talking and may stop laughing in public. Holly may reduce the number of presentations she volunteers for at work. She may miss out on acquiring clients and she may miss a promotion. If she is made redundant, Holly may struggle to find new work due to her reserved habits and lack of confidence in social situations. Prospective employers may be put off due to her appearance.

Also, losing one tooth can lead to losing another. Her teeth adjacent to the missing one have a higher risk of failure. She may need multiple days off work for further dental issues and treatment. In a few years, she may lose another tooth, and then another. The cycle goes on. Holly's confidence in her appearance reduces. If Holly were to lose all of her teeth, then she could fall into the statistic of people with all their teeth missing or dentures living approx. 9.8 years less than people with fixed teeth. What price would we put on that?

TOTAL LIFETIME COST= INCALCULABLE

HOLLY'S OPTION 2

Replace the missing tooth with a denture.

Initial cost NHS denture: £256.50 (UK 2019).

According to some statistics, dentures are being replaced on average every 5 years.

This is mainly due to bone shrinkage and the denture becoming too loose, or the denture being lost or broken.

If Holly lives an average age of 86-years, then purely in denture re-make charges, that is **£3,933.**

However, the presence of a denture increases the plaque in the mouth, increasing the risk of decay and gum disease to the adjacent teeth. So, let's imagine that Holly loses another tooth every 5 years. There are the additional costs of fillings, root canal treatments and then further extractions, bigger dentures and the lifetime cost of preventing and treating gum disease. Add to this the cost of time off work for dental pain and dental appointments, and the cost is much higher.

Plus, dentures have social implications for Holly similar to having missing teeth. Holly may reduce her input at work and withdraw socially due to the fear of her dentures moving or coming out during speaking and eating. In the same way as a missing tooth may impact Holly's job and social life, so does a denture. And again, if Holly were finally to lose all of her teeth, then she could fall into that statistic of people with all their teeth missing or dentures living 9.8 years less than people with fixed teeth. I would call that priceless.

TOTAL LIFETIME COST= Minimum £3,933 to INCALCULABLE

HOLLY'S OPTION 3

Replace the missing tooth with a dental bridge (supported by the remaining teeth on either side of the gap).

Initial cost: approx. £1,500. (estimated average private 3-unit bridge cost in the UK, 2019)

Statistically, a dental bridge may last on average 10 years. So, the number of repeat bridges throughout Holly's life could be another 4, so the overall long-term the cost could be **£7,500.**

However further to this, often the reason a bridge fails is this. The adjacent teeth are ground down to accommodate the bridge, and some research shows that approx. 30% of these teeth require root canal treatment due to the trauma of the bridge procedure. Root canal treatment weakens the teeth, leading to an increased risk of root fracture then bridge failure. So, every time a tooth fails, then the bridge fails. If another tooth is extracted, then the bridge gets longer, and the longevity of bridges reduces with increased span. This could continue until there are too many teeth missing and it is impossible to do any more bridges. So, in reality, it is unlikely that Holly would have 4 bridges. She would probably end up with many missing teeth and have to have a denture or several implants to replace them.

So, the costs are likely to be much higher than £7,500,

TOTAL LIFETIME COST: From £7,500 to INCALCULABLE

HOLLY'S OPTION 4

Replace the missing tooth with a single dental implant.

Initial cost approx. £2,400.

The bone is preserved. The adjacent teeth remain healthy. Holly goes back to normal after having her implant.

Holly remains confident socially and professionally. Her career is not impacted in any way. The implant is expected to last for life. Perhaps the implant-retained crown may become worn or chipped in several decades and may need replacing (approx. £800).

TOTAL LIFETIME COST: From £3,200

I believe that a key reason that patients do not opt for dental implants is the initial cost. We live in an immediate society.

However, it is time to look at the long-term picture for dental health, well-being and our lives.

It makes long-term financial sense to replace a missing tooth with a dental implant. They are great value for money.

Your quality of life is priceless.

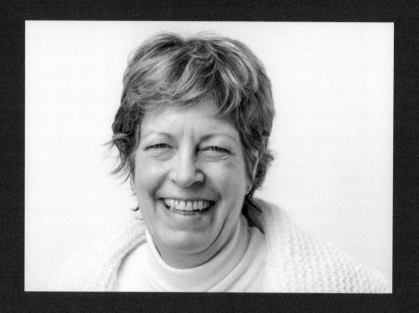

"I am so pleased with my new teeth and despite any initial concerns regarding procedure, costs, etc, consider it a valuable investment and has improved my confidence no end."

MRS LEEDHAM

"Implants gave me a second chance of having a good smile."

CHRIS BROOKES

FINALLY

I am often asked by friends, family and total strangers, "What would you do if you were me – if you were losing a tooth?"

If I had a failing tooth, before the tooth had even been extracted, this is what I would do.

I would have a consultation with a highly experienced implant surgeon and discuss replacing the failing tooth with an implant. The surgeon could plan a conservative extraction, minimising bone loss to maintaining optimum bone. In fact, the implant may be able to be placed directly into the socket at the time of extraction.

Each of us needs to weigh up the pros and cons of every decision we make personally at each point in our lives. Implants may or may not be the most appropriate option for you.

However, we have seen dental implants can breathe life back into smiles. They can give back our biting and chewing power, enabling us to eat everything that we want to. We can laugh, talk freely and even skydive without the fear of our dentures moving or falling out.

Dental implants give us a second chance of having a beautiful, confident smile.

SECTION 3

AT A GLANCE GUIDE TO YOUR OPTIONS

REPLACING A SINGLE MISSING TOOTH

OPTION 1:   DENTAL IMPLANT

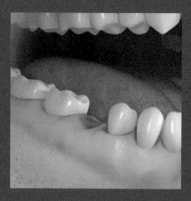

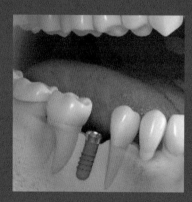

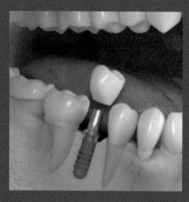

Advantages

- Fixed in place, not removeable
- Ability to bite into a crispy apple
- Preserves bone
- Good aesthetics
- Upper palate free of acrylic
- Keeps adjacent teeth healthy
- Ability to eat nutritious and fibrous diet
- Best life-time value

Disadvantages

- × Short-term: high initial cost

Average Time for Treatment

1-3 months (up to 6+ months with grafting)

Success Rate

Approx. 98%

Average Longevity

30+ years/lifetime

REPLACING A SINGLE MISSING TOOTH

OPTION 2:   DENTAL BRIDGE

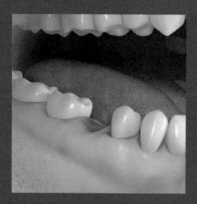

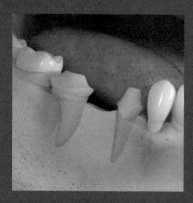

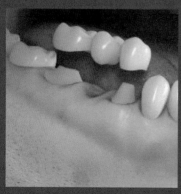

Advantages

- Fixed in place, not removeable
- Good biting ability, although significantly less than a dental implant
- Good initial aesthetics before on-going bone loss occurs
- Upper palate free of acrylic, unlike a denture

Disadvantages

- × Damage to adjacent teeth during preparation leading to high risk of nerve damage, root fracture and failure of the bridge.
- × Re-treatment can be complex and costly to replace a failed bridge
- × Does not preserves bone
- × Poor long-term aesthetics due to bone loss under the bridge, creating space
- × Food trapping under bridge over time, leading to increased risk of decay and gum disease

Cost

- Short-term: High initial cost
- Long-term: Very high ongoing costs including risk of root canal treatments, replacement bridges, and further complex treatment if further bridges are unfeasible.

Average Time for Treatment

1-3 weeks

Average Longevity

Approx. 10 years

REPLACING A SINGLE MISSING TOOTH

OPTION 3:   PARTIAL DENTURE

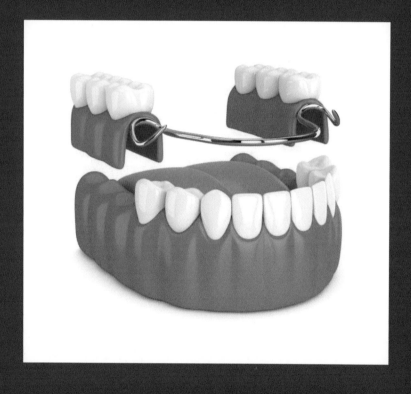

Advantages

- Cheap initially

Disadvantages

- × Not fixed in place, removeable
- × Increased risk of plaque build-up and increased risk of decay and gum disease of adjacent teeth
- × Does not preserves bone
- × Poor aesthetics
- × Food trapping under denture during eating
- × Large acrylic area in mouth
- × Leave out at night for disinfection
- × Becomes loose over time
- × High risk of social embarrassment
- × Reduced tasting ability if the palate is covered
- × Very low biting force, leading to reduced nutrition
- × Increased risk of medical diseases from reduced nutrition

Cost

- Short-term: low initial cost
- Long-term: very high due to
  - higher risk of treatment on adjacent teeth
  - multiple life-time replacement dentures
  - increased risks of health issues due to reduced nutrition

Average Time for Treatment

1 week

Longevity

Approx. 5 years

REPLACING A SINGLE MISSING TOOTH

OPTION 4:   LEAVE THE SPACE

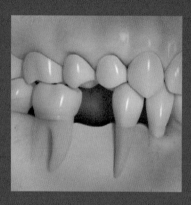

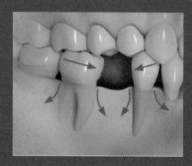

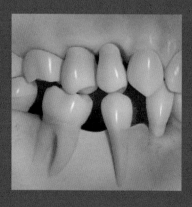

Advantages

☐ No cost short-term

Disadvantages

× Does not preserve bone
× Bone loss near adjacent teeth increases risk of decay, gum disease and further tooth loss
× Very poor aesthetics
× Adjacent teeth drift into the space, creating food-trapping, increasing risk of decay and gum disease
× Teeth above the space can drift downwards, increasing risk of bite problems, tooth fracture and jaw joint disorders
× High risk of social embarrassment
× Reduced biting force, leading to difficulty with nutrition
× Increased risk of stomach disorders due to partially-chewed foods.
× Increased risk of medical diseases due to reduced nutrition

Cost

- Short-term: low initial cost
- Long-term: Very high due to
    - higher risk of treatment needed to adjacent teeth
    - high cost of psychological impact due to embarrassment leading to increased risk of social isolation
    - health issues due to reduced nutrition.

Average Time for Treatment   Nil

OPTION 1:   FULL JAW DENTAL IMPLANT BRIDGE

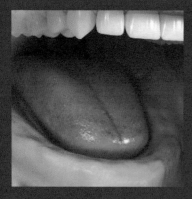

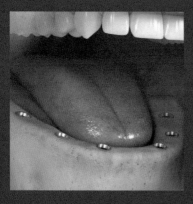

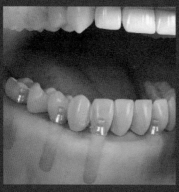

Advantages

- ☑ Fixed in place, not removeable
- ☑ Ability to bite into a crispy apple, increasing chance of maintaining a nutritious diet long term
- ☑ Preserves bone
- ☑ Good aesthetics
- ☑ Upper palate free of acrylic
- ☑ Best life-time value

Disadvantages

- × More difficult to clean than removeable options

Cost

- Short-term: highest initial cost
- Long-term: low

Average Time for Treatment

1-3 months (up to 6+ months with grafting)

Success Rate

98% average

Average Longevity

30+ years/lifetime

REPLACING ALL THE TEETH IN THE JAW

OPTION 2: IMPLANT-RETAINED DENTURE ON A BAR

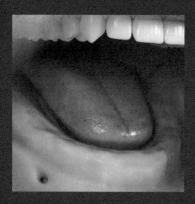

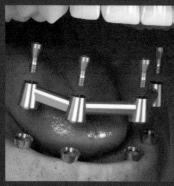

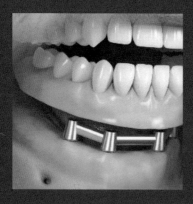

Advantages

- ☑ Fixed in place, however also removeable
- ☑ Ability to bite into a crispy apple
- ☑ Preserves bone
- ☑ Good aesthetics
- ☑ Upper palate free of acrylic
- ☑ Keeps adjacent teeth healthy
- ☑ Best life-time value
- ☑ Very high biting force, increasing nutrition
- ☑ Reduced risk of medical diseases due to ability for good nutrition

Disadvantages

- × Small acrylic area in mouth
- × Leave out at night for disinfection
- × Increased risk of oral fungal infections

Cost

- Short-term: higher initial cost
- Long-term: low cost

Average Time for Treatment

1-3 months (up to 6+ months with grafting)

Success rate

98% average

Average longevity

30+ years/lifetime

REPLACING ALL THE TEETH IN THE JAW

OPTION 3:   IMPLANT-RETAINED DENTURE ON LOCATOR-

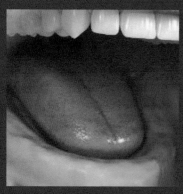

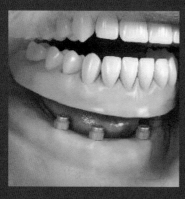

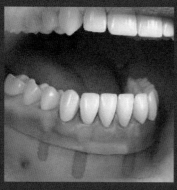

Advantages

- Fixed in place, however also removeable
- Good ability to bite
- Preserves bone
- Good aesthetics
- Great life-time value
- Very high biting force, leading to ability for great nutrition
- Reduced risk of medical diseases due to full nutrition

Disadvantages

- × Bite may not be strong enough to bite crispy apple
- × Removeable
- × Larger acrylic area in mouth, although much less than a full denture
- × Leave out at night for disinfection
- × Increased risk of oral fungal infections

Cost

- Short-term: higher initial cost
- Long-term: low

Average Time for Treatment

1-3 months (up to 6+ months with grafting)

Success Rate

98% average

Average Longevity

30+ years/lifetime

REPLACING ALL THE TEETH IN THE JAW

OPTION 4:   FULL DENTURE

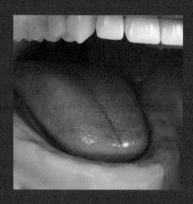

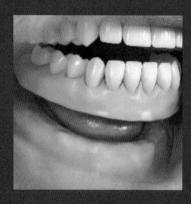

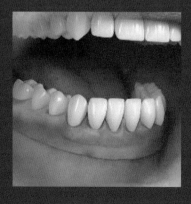

Advantages

- ☑ Cheap initially

Disadvantages

- ✕ Not fixed in place, removeable
- ✕ Increased risk of plaque build-up and increased risk of decay and gum disease of adjacent teeth
- ✕ Does not preserves bone
- ✕ Poor aesthetics
- ✕ Food trapping under denture during eating
- ✕ Large acrylic area in mouth
- ✕ Leave out at night for disinfection
- ✕ Becomes loose over time
- ✕ High risk of social embarrassment
- ✕ Reduced tasting ability if the palate is covered
- ✕ Increased risk of oral fungal infections
- ✕ Very low biting force, leading to reduced nutrition
- ✕ Increased risk of medical diseases due to reduced nutrition

Cost

- Short-term: low initial cost
- Long-term: very high due to
  - o higher risk of treatment on adjacent teeth
  - o multiple life-time replacement dentures
  - o increased risks of health issues due to reduced nutrition. Statistics show that denture wearers live 9.8 years on average less than those with fixed teeth

Average Time for Treatment   Approx. 4 weeks

Longevity   Approx. 5 years

REFERENCES

[1] Michael CG, Javid NS, Colaizzi FA, Gibbs CH. Biting strength and chewing forces in complete denture wearers. *J Prosthet Dent.* 1990 May; 63(5):549-53.

[2] van Kampen FM, van der Bilt A, Cune MS, Fontijn-Tekamp FA, Bosman F. Masticatory function with implant-supported overdentures. *J Dent Res.* 2004 Sep; 83(9):708-11.

[3] Allen PF, McMillan AS. A review of the functional and psychosocial outcomes of edentulousness treated with complete replacement dentures. *J Can Dent Assoc.* 2003 Nov; 69(10):662.

[4] Tsakos G, Herrick K, Sheiham A, Watt RG. Edentulism and fruit and vegetable intake in low-income adults. *J Dent Res. 2010 May; 89(5):462-7.*

[5] Locker D. *Community Dent Health.* 1992 Jun; 9(2):109-24.

[6] Locker D. The burden of oral disorders in a population of older adults. *Community Dent Health.* 1992 Jun; 9(2):109-24.

[7] Abnet CC, Qiao YL, Dawsey SM, Dong ZW, Taylor PR, Mark SD. Tooth loss is associated with increased risk of total death and death from upper gastrointestinal cancer, heart disease, and stroke in a Chinese population-based cohort. *International Journal of Epidemiology.* 2005;34(2):467–474. [**PubMed**]

[8] Sierpinska T, Golebiewska M, Dlugosz JW, Kemona A, Laszewicz W. Connection between masticatory efficiency and pathomorphologic changes in gastric mucosa. *Quintessence International.* 2007;38(1):31–37. [**PubMed**]

[9] Stolzenberg-Solomon RZ, Dodd KW, Blaser MJ, Virtamo J, Taylor PR, Albanes D. Tooth loss, pancreatic cancer, and Helicobacter pylori. *The American Journal of Clinical Nutrition.* 2003;78(1):176–181. [**PubMed**]

[10] Cleary TJ, Hutton JE. An assessment of the association between functional edentulism, obesity, and NIDDM. *Diabetes Care*. 1995;18(7):1007–1009. [**PubMed**]

[11] Medina-Solis CE, Perez-Nunez R, Maupome G, Casanova-Rosado JF. Edentulism among Mexican adults aged 35 years and older and associated factors. *American Journal of Public Health*. 2006;96(9):1578–1581. [**PMC free article**] [**PubMed**]

[12] Abnet CC, Qiao YL, Dawsey SM, Dong ZW, Taylor PR, Mark SD. Tooth loss is associated with increased risk of total death and death from upper gastrointestinal cancer, heart disease, and stroke in a Chinese population-based cohort. *International Journal of Epidemiology*. 2005;34(2):467–474. [PubMed]

[13] Völzke H, Schwahn C, Hummel A, et al. Tooth loss is independently associated with the risk of acquired aortic valve sclerosis. *American Heart Journal*. 2005;150(6):1198–1203. [PubMed]

[14] Takata Y, Ansai T, Matsumura K, et al. Relationship between tooth loss and electrocardiographic abnormalities in octogenarians. *Journal of Dental Research*. 2001;80(7):1648–1652. [PubMed]

[15] Okoro CA, Balluz LS, Eke PI, et al. Tooth loss and heart disease: findings from the Behavioral Risk Factor Surveillance System. *American Journal of Preventive Medicine*. 2005;29:50–56. [PubMed]

[16] de Pablo P, Dietrich T, McAlindon TE. Association of periodontal disease and tooth loss with rheumatoid arthritis in the US population. *Journal of Rheumatology*. 2008;35(1):70–76. [PubMed]

[17] Mollaoglu MN, Alpar R. The effect of dental profile on daily functions of the elderly. *Clinical Oral Investigations*. 2005;9(3):137–140. [PubMed]

[18] Mack F, Schwahn C, Feine JS, et al. The impact of tooth loss on general health related to quality of life among elderly Pomeranians: results from the study of health in Pomerania (SHIP-0) *International Journal of Prosthodontics.* 2005;18(5):414–419. [PubMed]

[19] Fisher MA, Taylor GW, Shelton BJ, et al. Periodontal disease and other nontraditional risk factors for CKD. *American Journal of Kidney Diseases.* 2008;51(1):45–52. [PubMed]

[20] Bucca C, Cicolin A, Brussino L, et al. Tooth loss and obstructive sleep apnoea. *Respiratory Research.* 2006;7:p. 8. [PMC free article] [PubMed]

[21] MacEntee MI, Glick N, Stolar E. Age, gender, dentures and oral mucosal disorders. *Oral Diseases.* 1998;4(1):32–36. [PubMed]

[22] Jainkittivong A, Aneksuk V, Langlais RP. Oral mucosal lesions in denture wearers. *Gerodontology.* 2010;27(1):26–32. [PubMed]

[23] Felton D, Cooper L, Duqum I, et al. Evidence-based guidelines for the care and maintenance of complete dentures: a publication of the American College of Prosthodontists. *Journal of the American Dental Association.* 2011;142(supplement 1):1S–20S. [PubMed]

[24] Owall et al, 2002; Int Journal of Prosthodontics, 15, 4 pg 371-378.

[25]**https://www.researchgate.net/publ**ication/7732409_Fate _of_vital_pulps_beneath_a_metal- ceramic_crown_or_a_bridge_retainer

[26] https://www.ncbi.nlm.nih.gov/pubmed/11856392

ACKNOWLEDGEMENTS

Thank you to our amazing patients who have selflessly shared their stories to help others. You are our inspiration.

Thank you to Steve Gibson, Kate Keating, Tim Steel, Sarah Chalk, Ric Fisher and Elle Ubhi for your time, attention to detail and delicately honest feedback.

A NOTE ABOUT THE AUTHORS

Dr Andrea Ubhi BChD founded her practice to focus patient care on dental implants and cosmetic dentistry in the heart of historic York. Graduating in dentistry in 1991, Andrea was a pioneer in cosmetic dentistry in the UK from the late 90s.

She was the youngest and first female to be named Dentist of the Year in 2005 at the Dental Awards, and she was named Employer of the Year in 2016 (Private Dentistry Awards). Her team was awarded National Team of the Year in 2018, 2017 & 2016 (the Dental Awards). www.andreaubhi.com

She is co-founder of Inspiring Women in Dentistry. Andrea is also chair of the charity, Asha Nepal, to which all profits from this book are donated, supporting survivors of trafficking and abuse. www.asha-nepal.org

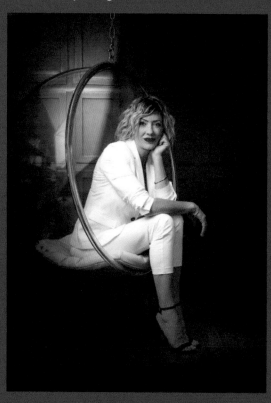

Dr Adam Glassford BChD Dip Con Sed(Ncle) Dip Imp Dent (RCS)(Eng.)(Adv cert) is the lead Dental Implant Surgeon at Andrea Ubhi Dentistry.

Dentists refer their patients to Adam for Dental Implants, Sedation & Cosmetic Dentistry from across the UK.

Adam qualified in Dentistry in 1996 from Leeds University and holds the Advanced Implant Diploma from the Royal College of Surgeons of England and also the Diploma in Conscious Sedation.

Adam is one of the leading dental implant providers of Swiss Straumann implants, the global manufacturer. Adam has placed over 6000 dental implants over the past 16 years and provides complex, advanced and simple implant treatments, including complex grafting procedures.

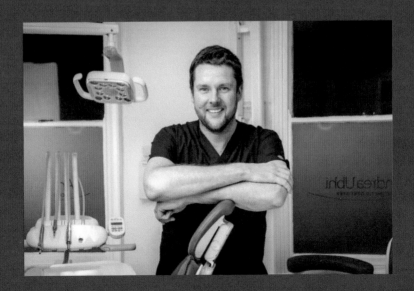

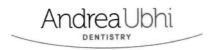

Printed in Poland
by Amazon Fulfillment
Poland Sp. z o.o., Wrocław

50478456R00140